DARK
VEILED
FACES

ISBN: 9798468968659

Editorial Advisor: Kat Harvey

Contents

AUTHOR'S NOTE

On completing the first draft of my book, I met a chap called Frith in the Pitmedden forest. As it turns out, we were at Heriot Watt at the same time, and though we never actually met, he said he remembered me as the guy that was always laughing. Anyway, he offered to give that early draft a read, and on doing so encouraged me to find a way to publish. When I saw him again last week, some seven months on, he told me that he'd reestablished contact with his sister, who has epilepsy – after not having spoken to her for many years – and he thanked me for opening his eyes to the effects of epilepsy medications. I know that I'm taking a chance by opening this can of worms, for there are some who will not understand, but no matter what happens now, my gamble has already paid off.

I've decided to dedicate my book to those who supported me when no one else would: my brother David, Mum and Dad, and Manuel – and, of course, to my best friend, Bobby McGee.

FOREWORD

Though they can be physical, the detrimental side effects with anticonvulsants are far more likely to be behavioural. Whereas an allergic reaction can, and should, be easily spotted, changes in an individual's character are far less likely to be attributed to the drugs – especially where no effort is made to monitor their mental health. Arrogance is a common side effect with drugs that animate the mind, but though my egotism has nurtured a succession of dismal failures, arrogance was far from the worst. They say you can't recognise madness in yourself, and that was certainly true for me. But though I can look back now and see the insanity, I want others to judge for me, as now the arrogance has abated, I am less sure of myself *(definitely a change for the better)*. Having exhausted all other options in trying to make a success of my life, I've decided to tell my story, in the hope it will inspire change.

I did have a line edit done, but though accepting most of the corrections to grammar and syntax, I rejected some of the edits; not because they were bad, but because they didn't sound like me. Given this will almost certainly be the only thing I publish in my life, I want it to be a reflection of my individuality – brain damage included – so please forgive my unusual writing style.

I have exhibited some extraordinary behaviour over the years, in part, down to a brain lesion, but much more profoundly – anticonvulsant drugs. Diagnosed at twelve years old, and of the first generation to be effectively treated for epilepsy, I spent thirty years finding a drug that would control the seizures and another ten finding one where the adverse side effects are less debilitating than the disease itself. Though I'm not looking to attribute blame, knowing every doctor that treated me did so with good intent, there are serious shortcomings in the way we monitor the effects of anticonvulsants on individual patients, and I will try to expose them here.

Before getting underway, I should point out that the detail is drawn entirely from memory, so there will be some ambiguity. The best analogy I can draw is with the effects of alcohol. When I used to wake in the morning after a booze up, with little or no recollection of the previous night's goings on; after a few drinks, it all came flooding back. The way that we think and access memories is dependent on our state of mind. My mind was heavily influenced by epilepsy medications – its chemical balance changing whenever I was switched from one drug to another, impairing access to memories and often leaving me unable to recognise people from my past.

Several of my stories sound vain, unappealing and redundant, not enhancing my image in any way. Things I wouldn't have included were this a work of fiction. But this is not a fantasy, rather it is a chronicle of excessive behaviour, persistent failure and, most importantly, an example of how anticonvulsants can ruin a life.

Though some may seem irrelevant to my battle with mental health, the trials and tribulations recorded here are the only comparative measure I have to show how each of the drugs affected my personality. I am naturally (when not influenced by drugs or alcohol) an introvert, preferring not to develop close ties with others, and so, perhaps ironically, there have been many brief acquaintances. I've done my best to include only the most relevant so as not to confuse, but keep in mind, this is an examination of my character and how it was contorted by drugs, so the other characters are incidental.

I have recorded everything exactly as I remember it. Including strong language, perverse behaviour and delusional rambling.

I considered dialing things down, so as to maintain a modicum of good taste, but decided that would simply obscure the reality, so batten down the hatches.

Comments in italics are based on what I know now rather than what I believed at the time. They include clarification where my understanding has changed, and my insights on writing the book.

INTRODUCTION

Born in Lerwick, Shetland, on 31 July 1967, Mum tells me that I had a convulsion of sorts as an infant, but as there was no recurrence, it was forgotten about. My first memories would be of living at Dore Holm in Urafirth, Shetland, where my parents worked for the Co-Op, with Dad driving a Co-Op van serving crofters and small villages in the area and Mum running the shop. Memories here are limited to two old wrecks on the beach – seeming enormous and awe-inspiring at the time, only later to be realised as the remains of two very small rowing boats – and the tinned strawberries with Bird's Dream Topping I got each day from our elderly neighbours Neenie and Vera (mother and daughter).

At four and a half, we moved to a new council house in Brae, and to my utter dismay, school, by far preferring the wooden packing case Dad rescued from a dumpster and brought home for me to play with in the back garden. Mum tells me that all the kids would come over to play in the box – one day a boat, the next a truck; indeed, it was perfectly suited to any and all adventures. I won't waste more time on these early years as, though happy and idyllic in their setting, they are not important to this story.

The next big step would be, in the summer of 1975 at eight years old, moving from Shetland to Pitmedden Farm just north of Auchtermuchty on the Scottish mainland. It was by far the most beautiful place I've ever lived – a large farm cottage on the side of a hill that overlooks a glen enclosed by the Pitmedden forest. The view from the house stretched far into the distance, including the Lomond hills in all their majesty. Dad managed two adjoining farms – Pitmedden and Raemore – giving me the freedom to do pretty much as I pleased. Driving tractors at every opportunity, helping with the feeding and bedding of the animals, and working the fields, tossing hay bales up into stacks four high, *pretty good for an eight-year-old*. With the strings cutting into my hands, it was bloody sore, but there was no point wearing leather gloves as they would be ruined in a day. In 1976, with the weather scorching, I was harassed to the point of madness by flies, but I stuck at it, hoping to impress Dad, for he could throw the bales further than any of the workers that came up from the village, and I wanted to be like him.

The tatties were just as hard, though I managed to wangle some shifts driving the tractor or emptying baskets into the trailer, both of which were much easier than bending down and picking tatties from the ground. I remember feeling some considerable guilt at watching the men do the easy work and leaving the much harder ground-picking to the women.

Earlier that summer, Grandad Woode and I saw a Chopper bike in the Halfords bike shop in Glenrothes. He said he'd pay for it there and then, and I could pay him back with my tattie money. Though he ended up saying I needn't bother when the tatties were done, I insisted, though a little reluctantly, and the debt was repaid.

With a speedometer that went up to 40 mph, a limit that, of course, had to be reached. On its maiden trip, I took it to the top of the steep hill that led to Raemore and pedalled with all my might. On reaching 30 mph I changed up to third gear, and as the needle touched forty, the bike went into a speed wobble, flipped into the air, and I skidded down the road on my nose. Fortunately, there were no bad injuries, just some scrapes on my hands and face, and more importantly, the bike survived. Taking it to my workshop to assess the damage, I covered a couple of scratches on the seat with black boot polish, and no one was any the wiser. Pretty much the entire four years we lived at Pitmedden were spent outdoors doing stuff, whether that be "working", building gang huts, rolling down hills inside an old water tank in turns with David, my younger brother, scrambling with our bikes or building "stuff" in my workshop.

Grandad would tell us bedtime stories whenever they came over for the weekend, Br'er Rabbit and Br'er Fox then Sherlock Holmes. In the years to come, he made me a wooden chess table with drawers, lined in velvet, to hold the hand-painted plaster of paris pieces, and taught me to play. Granny Woode was my favourite grandparent though, for she was so easy-going and matter-of-fact. Having walked five miles to school each day as a child, brought up on a Shetland croft, I think she found the modern world a little confusing. On one occasion, many years later, when on a weekend drive to Stirling, David called Dad on his mobile, and Granny turned to Mum to ask, "How did David know we were here?"

I didn't have much contact with my father's parents for they lived in Norway when I was very young, and although they stayed a short time at Lauriston near Falkirk before moving down south to Middlesborough, I never really took to them for they were very religious.

Then there was school. Here, my main memories are of sports. Though not all that good, I was strong, and with my classmates sadly lacking, I tended to win all the events on school sports day. Indeed, the only one in my class who could compete with me in running was Davina, or Venus as she insisted on being addressed. She was an out-and-out tomboy and might well have beaten me had we ever raced head-to-head. On occasion, she would arrive at Pitmedden on her Chopper, and we'd race our bikes or something of the like.

When playing football for the school against Newburgh, we got a penalty, and Billy, the class hardman, grabbed the ball to take it. Given it was me that was fouled, and I was captain, I picked up the ball and said I was taking it. Billy got really angry and started shouting at me, but I took the penalty and, of course, missed. Billy was substituted and subsequently dropped in our next match. No more was said of the matter, but a few days later, Scot, my best friend at primary school, asked if I was coming to the fight. And though not all that interested, I went anyway.

When we arrived at the fire station, Colin, a friend of Billy's from the class below ours, confronted me, "I want a fight."

Taken by surprise I asked, "Why? I thought we were mates."

"I want to be able to say I'm harder than you."

"You can say you're harder than me if you like, I'm not going to fight just so I can say I'm harder than you."

And that was that. I walked away to half-hearted cheers as he celebrated his victory – the waiting crowd seeming a wee bit disappointed.

Though I wasn't all that interested in academic stuff while at primary school, I did enjoy being on stage. First time up, reciting "The Four Winds" by Sandy Thomas Ross together with Venus at the school concert, reading two verses each. The next year playing Delaney in "Delaney's Donkey", and finally, I was the father in "Albert and the Lion", where my son, Albert, was eaten by a lion, and on complaining to the zoo, I stressed, "He was in his Sunday best too." All great fun, but that was the extent of my dalliance with stardom.

Though not having any full seizures while at Pitmedden, at ten years old I did have an absence seizure of sorts when building hay in the barn at Raemore. And throughout my time at primary school, I occasionally felt "head-light", thinking that meant a click followed by a sharp flash of pain through my skull when turning my head too quickly to the left. Having heard my elders talk about feeling head-light on getting up too quickly, though very painful, I accepted this as normal.

Near the end of my last year at primary school, Dad's boss, a drunken Orcadian, decided to sell the farms. This might have been a huge blow, but luckily, a position as head stockman had just become vacant only a few miles away on a large estate belonging to Major Russell, a founder of the Tullis Russell Paper Mill. It was a beautiful place down in the lowlands, so less of a view, but other than that, it was perfect.

EPILIM

On to Bell Baxter High School where my expectations of a far more interesting and diverse learning environment were soon dashed. My registration class was A9, the lowest of the French-taking classes. In my first week, Stewart, one of my old friends from primary school, came running up to me in the corridor, while we stood waiting for class, and started punching me, shouting something about me telling everyone I was harder than him. Having no idea what he was talking about, my lack of retaliation singled me out as an easy target for bullies in the year to come. Stewart told me years later that a boy from Cupar called Simi had admitted he'd lied about what I'd said as he wanted to see if Stewart could take me, so he'd beaten up Simi but felt lousy because he'd not had the courage to come to me and apologise.

Toward the middle of my first term (first year – 1979), on my way to school, I woke up in the back of an ambulance after having had a grand-mal seizure. Apparently, the double-decker school bus had almost capsized as it passed with all the kids at the windows trying to see what had happened. Feeling sick to my stomach on being told it was epilepsy, partly because there had been a girl at primary school with epilepsy and all my friends said her mum was a witch, but more importantly because it ruled out driving – a dream that would be shattered time and time again in the years to come. I told friends at school I'd been hit by a car. Then after another public seizure, when Scot said it had really been a fit at the bus stop, I angrily insisted otherwise as if believing denial would somehow stop epilepsy ruining my life. As the rest of first year dragged by, I was started on an epilepsy medication called Epilim, and though there were no obvious ill effects with the drug, I became very nervous of girls and was sure this was a side effect.

On reaching second year, things improved enormously. I found a good friend in Malcolm, and my classmates were a much nicer lot, on dropping from A9 to B10 and out of the French classes. When a bully called Gary started tormenting one of my classmates from primary school, I decided to put a stop to it. Malcolm and me met Gary in a quiet corridor one day and told him to stop bullying Robin, and he did. Then one lunchtime, when waiting to go back into class, me and a couple of others were jumping up and trying to touch the ceiling, when Gary grabbed my hair and pulled me down. Turning with natural instinct, I punched him in the face. There were cheers from the girls as the blood started pouring from his nose. When the teacher arrived, we were taken to see the deputy head, Mr Dick. He asked me to explain what had happened, and I told him exactly. He said we should stand in line with no jumping when waiting for our teacher, then he asked Gary if what I'd said was correct. When he said yes, Mr Dick told Gary to go the nurse and sent me back to class. It may have helped that I was good at maths, and he was our maths teacher.

Then one day, Malcolm's mum arrived in our history class to pick him up. I later learnt that she'd split with his father, and they were leaving the area. The following week, Gary came up to me and said, "What are you going to do now your big friend is gone?" To which I replied, "If I remember rightly, I didn't need his help last time," and he backed off. The next week, he was moved to another class after his mother complained to the rector that I'd been bullying him – an accusation that was never officially put to me by the school, though on telling me, our English teacher seemed glad to be rid of him.

I really enjoyed second year, particularly art as we had a great teacher. There was a very painful four-of-the-belt from our history teacher for writing a lot of squiggles instead of words in my jotter when we were supposed to be doing a written assignment in class – but other than that, it was a good laugh. I even got to take the prettiest girl in school, Karen Smith, to the school dance. While desperately trying to work up the courage to ask her to dance, Derek, another boy from my class who had a date with Karen's friend, grabbed my hands, and we started dancing around the floor like a pair of idiots. And that was the end of that – a brutally disappointing night.

Now for *Joe* ... *Joe* was an old trapper. I had great respect for *Joe*, believing him to be highly intelligent and extremely kind. Having known *Joe* for what seemed like many years, for one so young, I had come to see him as a man I would want to emulate. Then one day, he took out some porn mags and said he'd show me what a blow job was. I was very uncomfortable, but I let him do it, did not orgasm and refused to do the same for him. At somewhere between twelve and fourteen years old, it only happened that one time, and I stopped going to see him thereafter. I would rather not have included this rotten business, but I have to unearth all the skeletons or my story will not be complete. He betrayed my trust that day, and there is a chance that is why I never allow myself to commit to relationships – or maybe this was nothing more than a sordid coincidence, and I was always destined for the single life. Whatever the truth, he is long-since dead and it's better forgotten.

During my first two years at high school, I was having seizures every two to five months, so relatively infrequently, most often at night, though occasionally in the early morning. They were grand-mal, starting with my head turning to the left and eyes staring over my shoulder before going into convulsions. On waking, deadly tired with my tongue badly bitten, I would sleep for twenty-four hours and still feel tired with a sickly stomach for another twenty-four before enduring several days of painful eating while my tongue healed.

A consultant once told me to imagine there being a volatile electrical connection in my brain. As long as that link remains intact everything is fine, but when the current falls too low, the connection breaks and, after a time, charge builds up at either side of the break, until eventually, there is a spark, and the connection reforms. But this surge of energy is too much for the brain to handle, so it's thrown into seizure. The objective is to stop the initial break by invigorating the part of the brain that's affected. My trouble over the years has been in finding a drug that invigorates the problem area and not the rest of the brain. This will become more evident later.

Interestingly, I was never long depressed after recovering from the initial shock of a seizure, and this was recently explained to me by Dave, a psychiatric nurse back in the days when ECT (electroconvulsive therapy) was commonly used. Apparently, ECT induces a grand-mal seizure, only the patient is given drugs to paralyse the muscles and stop convulsions, thereby preventing tongue-biting and exhaustion. Most often used to treat severe depression, the treatment effectively reboots the brain. Hence my unexpected upbeat demeanour post-seizure.

EPILIM & PHENYTOIN

Before entering third year at Bell Baxter, my prescription was changed from Epilim to both Epilim and Phenytoin. I don't remember this change making me feel all that different, though I did feel a little drowsy at first. It did not reduce seizure activity but possibly kept things in check.

On a lighter note, I will take a break from school and tell you more about home. There were four farms on Major Russell's estate – Lower Rossie, Kilwhiss, Meadowwells and Cadham (the site of the paper mill). We lived at Lower Rossie, next to the Major's mansion. It was a long cottage with three large downstairs bedrooms and two smaller bedrooms in the attic, one of which was used as a billiards room, and the other for darts and gathering dust. There was a big steading with a good-sized byre, sheds for hay and grain and plenty of room for my own workshop. Away from the steading, there were miles of beautiful walks stretching out into the bog – a fair expanse of land still too wet to be farmed after draining, this being the domain of the gamekeeper and his pheasants.

One winter, when it was cold enough for a deep frost, David and me decided to go round to the pond at the back of the gamie's house with our bikes. It was hard-frozen in the centre, but the gamie had driven round the edge with his tractor to let the pheasants get water, and though partially refrozen, that ice was too thin. Not to be deterred, we threw our bikes onto the thick ice and jumped across. After a considerable time tearing around, I calculated that, taking a run at it, the bike would be going fast enough to skim over the thin ice. So I went to the opposite side of the pond, readied myself and pedalled with all my might … On hitting the thin ice, there was a loud cracking sound, and I plummeted downward. David immediately burst out laughing and valiantly offered his hand only to land in the water beside me. We laughed hysterically before succumbing to the cold. Now far too cold to cycle, we picked up our bikes and walked painfully home. I've never felt so cold in my life and, to this day, don't know how we made it back.

Back to Rossie. There was a small, enclosed garden at the far side of the gamie's storage barn, about thirty yards from the house, and it was here that Dad built a lean-to greenhouse and summerhouse. The summerhouse was a single room built with wood from old packing cases and faced with strips of bark; it looked like a log cabin. There was a lawn with flowerbeds and rockeries, and even a small pond with a fountain, so we could always hear running water. The perfect retreat from the world.

There were another two larger lawns between the house and a small burn that trickled down the far side of a dirt track. David spent many an hour there catching eels and taking them back upstream for release, only to rush back down and catch them again. One Christmas when cycling this track with no hands and zipping up my new biker's jacket, my front wheel hit the dyke, and I flew over the handlebars down a six-foot drop into the burn with the Chopper landing on top of me. On regaining my composure, I heard gales of laughter as Mum, Dad and David seemed unable to catch their breath.

Now to what is probably the stupidest thing I've ever done, and I'm going to attribute this to Phenytoin numbing my brain, for I need an excuse. While working with Dad and Uncle Ken at The Clink (Ken's farm) building hay bales into the steading, Ken turned the bale elevator off, and I decided to grab the belt between the engine and the pulleys just before it completely stopped, on the last chug, to see if I could stop it manually. As a result, the fingers on my left hand were pulled between a pulley and the belt, taking the tip off my little finger and the nails off the rest. Could this be why they say "do not operate heavy machinery" when on sedatives?

As a child, I did lots of stupid stuff, like forgetting to close the slide door on the barley trailer, which left a tell-tale trail of barley from the combine to the barn. Then leaving the imprint of the tractor's grill in the corrugated-iron shed door when misjudging stopping distance while towing that same, still heavy, trailer. I didn't get a lot of tractor work on the farm thereafter, but it's hard to imagine a better upbringing, perhaps explaining my aversion to school.

With pretty good grades in second year, good enough to be the only one in my class to get a "blue sheet" – a sheet that came with our exam results, meaning that I would return to the upper classes – hating languages, my choice was between technical and science. Understanding that biology would mean cutting up frogs, and not prepared to kill a creature for no good reason, I went with the technical option which included physics and chemistry anyway. A huge mistake, for there were a number of boys who didn't get blue sheets whose parents insisted they were placed in the upper classes, and the school agreed with the understanding they took technical. Reunited with the buffoons from my first year and a few other unsavoury characters, my third and fourth years were not nearly as much fun as they might have been.

When hearing that Edie, a quiet and submissive lad, had given Simi a good hiding rather than put up with his abuse, I was well impressed, until a few days later when Simi came running up the path and hit me with a couple of punches looking to restore his reputation. On avoiding a third, I saw a teacher we called Bamber running toward us, so I held on to Simi and let him continue punching until Bamber grabbed him.

I told Bamber I had no idea what Simi's problem was, he'd just started hitting me, which Simi could not deny for Bamber had seen everything. Simi was dragged off for punishment, and I continued on my way down the path to where my best mate Keith was waiting. The next day Simi appeared again as we walked down the playing fields, shouting that it wasn't over, and he intended to "finish the job". I laughed, saying, "Fuck off, McClelland!" He did, and as a result, fewer called me Salmon or Pike thereafter.

I was also called Salmon at the five-aside football we played in a nearby village called Collessie. I now like to think I was the "king of the fish", but back then, my big eyes and substantial nose seemed the more likely explanation. We played five-aside football every Saturday, something I truly loved. Dad would often come along, for he was a great player, having played for Shetland and only missing out on being signed for Raith Rovers (in the top-flight of Scottish football at the time) because he was too old when they spotted him. One Saturday, when David broke his wrist diving to save my shot – his arm caught between ball and post – I ran back up the field and told him to, "Get up and get on with it!" The poor lad was eventually taken to the hospital to get a stookie. I guess I wasn't the most sympathetic of characters.

Then there was our big day. We got to the final of the indoor five-a-side North-East Fife district championships where we came up against Cupar, a place hundreds of times larger than Collessie. With Cupar 2–0 up at half-time, as we stood ready to start the second half, I told our captain, Big Lop, to tap the ball to me rather than me to him as we had at the restarts after each of their goals. When he asked me why, I said, "Just do it and see what happens."

He did, and I kicked the ball straight up the middle, running as fast as I could after it, tapping it to the left while still going forward and just managing to get my right foot across the ball to flick it back into the top right corner of the net before it ran into the box and out of play. A few minutes later, Big Lop got a cracking goal with a great shot from distance, and in the last minute, Maurice (our left back) scored the winner.

My third and fourth years at school were pretty dull. Other than the aforementioned incident with Simi, nothing much out of the ordinary happened. Mum and Dad got me a tutor for maths – Mrs Grant, a lovely old lady and fantastic teacher. We covered the syllabus pretty quickly, and apparently, she told Mum I was a natural talent.

In class after our maths prelims, our teacher read out the results starting with "A: band five, Anthony Doull, A: band four, Keith Stenhouse …" At first, I thought band one was best, then as he continued down through the Bs and Cs, I realised band five must be the highest. But there was a certain guilt in knowing Keith got his band four without the benefit of a tutor and so should really have been top. One of the buffoons from my first-year class said, "What?" when my name was read out, and a very pretty girl came up to congratulate me as we left the class. I felt eight feet tall.

Only really socialising with Keith in those years, we played billiards in school or at the farm, and snooker at our local club in Kirkcaldy. I preferred the shorter five- or six-foot tables, finding it hard to focus on the balls when playing a full-size twelve-foot table, because of astigmatism particularly in my left eye. Studying was not a priority, but I did okay in my O grade exams with three As, three Bs, two Cs and an F. Where F was for English – most definitely my Achilles heel.

In the fifth year, I took five Highers: maths, physics, technical drawing, engineering science and metalwork, and O grade art. Keith and me took charge of the billiards room because we were the best players and wanted the best table. One day fairly early in the year, there was an argument with a boy from Cupar. A nasty piece of work, he was always being catty and putting people down. Facing up to him, walking forward as he stepped back, and brushing his cheeks with fairly gentle punches, I felt really stiff as if for some reason unable to control my swing, likely something to do with adrenaline. Anyway, he didn't hit back, and the bell rang for class.

The next day, he came back into the billiard room, told me it wasn't over and I hadn't hurt him. Remembering how well it worked with Simi, I said, "Fuck off, Brown," then, "I said – fuck off, Brown." and he left, declaring it wasn't over. A few days later, as we entered the billiard room, there were two guys, one built like a brick shithouse, holding the best billiard table.

I said, "This is our table," and we took it from them.

The big guy said, "You'll pay for that."

Dismissing his threat with a "whatever" I started our game.

The next thing I know, I'm lying on the floor, watching Keith ask the guy why he'd done that.

On regaining my composure, I wasn't sure what to do, but decided I had to hit back.

As I got to my feet, he turned to look at me, and I hit him square on the chin with a right hook. His legs failed, and he fell to the floor. Just catching himself with the side of the billiard table, he looked at me and said, "I certainly wasn't expecting that," then pulled himself to his feet and countered with two or three punches, knocking me unconscious again.

This time, on coming round, I asked Keith where the guy had gone, and he said they'd just left.

I got to my feet, picked up a billiard cue, and muttering, "Quite a hardy cunt," I continued with our game.

Later that week, while walking up the school playing fields alone, I saw the same two across on the path heading down to the gate. One of them shouted, "Alright, Tony."

I shouted, "Alright, boys," and they waved back.

I wish I could remember the big guy's name, for this was the best thing that could possibly have happened as nobody gave me any shit thereafter. The guys called me Tony or Big Doull, and the girls treated me like I was the berries.

Of course, I was interested in girls, particularly a very pretty, petite blonde with blue-green eyes and brightly coloured stockings – a typical French maiden called Maria Ladelle who sat with me in art class. But even then, I was way too shy to do anything about it. My love life was more of a fantasy than anything else.

When it came to schoolwork, I really didn't pay much heed in fifth year, far more interested in playing billiards and snooker and daydreaming about girls. Winning the billiards singles and doubles titles was little recompense for failing all my Highers. I did get an A for O grade art, but because I couldn't drive or do any jobs that involved working with machinery, I had to stay on for sixth year. Unfortunately, Mrs Grant didn't teach Higher maths, so we asked my teacher at school, coincidentally the same Bamber who "saved" me from Simi.

On retaking all the fifth year Highers, plus Higher art, I was not at all impressed with Bamber's teaching when compared to Mrs Grant, but I did scrape a C this time round, as was true for all my Highers. As for O grade English, having failed that again in fifth year with an E, Mum and Dad got me a tutor. After a few weeks, he decided I had absolutely no ability in English and prepared a model answer to the reading question in the exam for me to learn off by heart, which I did and got an A.

To my great relief, I'd got a conditional offer from Strathclyde University reading physics, with the condition I pass O grade English. Knowing this had to be a mistake, having previously failed all my Highers, I accepted the offer on passing English. They did contact me to say there had been a mistake, but they would honour the offer given I'd passed all six Highers.

Before heading off to uni, my prescription for Phenytoin was doubled, with Epilim left as before, so memories of my time in Glasgow are thin on the ground. On arrival, I was allocated a shared room – because of the epilepsy – at the Baird Hall of Residence on Sauchiehall Street, but I can't for the life of me remember my roommate's name. My only memory of classes, though sure I attended the majority, was asking the lecturer a question at the end of one of our first physics lectures. When another student reeled off a very complicated answer, the lecturer agreed and turned to me to ask if I'd understood. Though having no idea what he was talking about, I said yes so as not to look stupid. Other than that day, I have no memory of lecturers or even the look of the campus. My second memory would be playing a racing car game at a small arcade next to the Baird Hall, getting all the top scores as TON, where on the last game, the engine noise got so loud everyone came over to see what was happening. I punched in TON as the new top score, got up and left. I did make a friend in physics class, a guy called Locwa Chu whose grandfather owned a chip shop in Glasgow, and we took a trip down to see Aunt Daphne in Southsea during one of our term breaks, but that's a very hazy recollection.

After some weeks in Glasgow, my roommate called my parents to tell them I seemed very drowsy and was unable to sit up in bed. It was later determined the Phenytoin dose was much too high, so it was reduced back to the previous prescription.

Other than developing a love for cheeseburger and raw onions, copying a load of tapes from the Baird Hall's record library and waking in hospital a few times after seizures, that is pretty much all I can remember of my time at Strathclyde. I did consider asking others, my aunt for example, but decided this account should be based primarily on my memories as that will reveal more of how these medications affected me.

Failing my first year at Strathclyde, though I don't remember sitting any exams, I then applied to take a degree in Applicable Mathematics at the Dundee College of Technology and was accepted on the grounds that there had been a problem with my medication while in Glasgow. I'm afraid my attitude toward learning wasn't great in Dundee, spending more time partying, playing snooker and propping up bars than in class.

I moved into catered lodgings on Arbroath Road in Dundee, including bed, breakfast and dinner, which I could take to my room when late in. I hadn't been there long before being asked to move out. It would seem my tardiness, constant drinking and the mess in my room, where they often found dirty plates under my bed, was not what they were looking for in a house guest.

Next to one of the halls of residence where five of us shared a flat, already running low on funds, I got a part-time job at a nearby Tesco. I enjoyed my time there, serving cheese and cold meat, but after a couple of months, having had a seizure on the job, they decided it was no longer safe for me to use the meat-slicing machine, so I quit.

On getting an F for an economics essay and telling my tutor I'd used a dictionary, which I had not, it was upgraded to C – for dyslexia was now considered a disability – but this infuriating inability to communicate ideas on paper continued to stifle my progress. *Though my spelling is much improved since taking up crosswords a few years ago, writing is still very difficult.*

I only recall attending one party. It was at the flat of a girl called Denise, her initials being DEC, I remember because that was the name of the mainframe computer at the college. She was really hot with short, jet-black hair, high cheek bones, very dark – almost black – eyes, and she was always smiling. I fancied her big style, but on getting drunk, I was sick and had to head home. She came to me the following day to apologise for her boyfriend giving me the pint of urine that made me sick. I didn't remember that but decided to steer clear thereafter, so I guess he achieved his goal.

Spending more of my time playing snooker, I was getting pretty good as my eyes now seemed better able to focus on the long shots. One day, an elderly guy came over and said there was a player from another club who wanted to challenge me to a match, best of three. He explained the stake was this guy's giro (his fortnightly benefits cheque), and he was going to cover the bet.

I won the first game but was behind at the end of the second with only pink and black left. They were at opposite ends of the table, both tight on the end cushions, about eighteen inches from diagonally opposite pockets. The white was next to the black, leaving a dangerous shot, very difficult to get safe and almost impossible to pot. Deciding my best course was to pot myself out of trouble, I hit the white with loads of side spin, so it arced its way up the table, caught the cushion just before hitting the pink, and spun toward the pocket so making the pot. But because I'd hit the ball so hard, it went all the way around the table leaving exactly the same shot on the black into the opposite corner. I sunk the pot again to win game and match, and my opponent signed his giro, slammed it on the table and walked off. The fellow who won the bet said his pal thought there was no chance I'd get the pink, though he'd said I would, but even he didn't think I'd pot the black as well. Please forgive this indulgence, I promise there will be no more talk of snooker shots.

Soon after, *Joe* made his second appearance. This *Joe* was a man in his mid-forties that I occasionally played snooker with at the Masters Snooker Club. On the night in question, we'd played a few games before he started talking about fitness and how strong I looked. He said there were chest expanders at his flat I could have if I fancied building up my chest muscles. In retrospect, that might seem like a strange thing for him to suggest, but I was young and naïve, and a little drunk thanks to him having bought a fair number of pints. When we got back to his flat, he invited me in, handed me the chest expanders to try and went to the fridge for two more beers. I tried the chest expanders but could only get them about two-thirds open, so he took them from me to show how it was done. With his jacket off, now wearing a white T-shirt, he was very muscular and quite intimidating. Handing me the beer, he went over to the bedside cabinet in his studio flat, grabbed something from a drawer, and turned to me saying he'd got it when in the navy as he pressed a button on its side and a blade flicked out.

Getting worried, I said, "I'd better get off as I have an early class."

He said, "No, you can stay here tonight."

I eventually agreed and undressed before getting into his bed, lying facing away from him. Keeping my ass tight shut for I would rather have been stabbed than raped, I waited for him to finish pleasuring himself and asked if I could go. He said yes of course, but I was not to say anything of this to the people at the snooker club. I told him I would never say anything of this to anyone, he could be sure of that.

I walked the three miles uptown to the halls and immediately took a shower. The next day, stopping by the Masters Snooker Club to pick up my cue, I never returned.

To this day, I cannot understand why I undressed for him. I can only assume it was the combination of Epilim, Phenytoin and alcohol that left me fearing for my life. Fear can be a hellish torment when it's exacerbated by drugs like these. The only analogy I can bring is with the shock felt on learning a loved one is dying.

On reaching the end of my first year at Dundee, once again having failed all my exams, Dr Roberts at the Dundee Royal Infirmary decided to do a brain scan (angiogram) because he felt the nature of my seizures, the way my head turned just before onset, suggested there might be a brain lesion. The scan showed a vascular malformation which would eventually need surgery. With a letter from my doctor confirming this, I was able to persuade the college to let me resit first year. Not long after the restart, on meeting with Mr Varma, the brain surgeon at DRI, we agreed surgery could wait until I'd completed the repeat year.

On moving to Whitfield to share a multi-storey flat with Neil, a drinking pal from my first-year class, he told me Whitfield had the highest murder rate in Europe, and that the year before, when the guy in the top flat threw his washing machine out the window onto a panda car parked outside the building, there had been a collection among the residents of Whitfield to get him a new one.

The repeat year went pretty much as the first. I joined the Victoria Road snooker club – from where my racing bike was pinched after only a week of leaving it at the top of the stairwell at the entrance to the club – again I spent the majority of my time on the green baize. I can barely remember attending any classes and have no recollection of classmates. My two most prominent memories this time round are of feeling faint and almost passing out when climbing stairs somewhere in the college, the same stairwell each time.

I do remember Neil rescuing a ginger kitten and Mum coming to Dundee to pick it up and take it back to the farm. She said he'd been sick in his cardboard box in the back of the car, somehow clawed his way out, jumped up onto the back of her seat and sat on her shoulder with his cold, wet, sticky tail wrapped round her neck. Higgins, as he became known, turned out to be a fine addition to the family.

21

Early in July of 1988, at the brain surgery pre-op, I asked Mr Varma to quantify the risks. He explained there was maybe a two per cent chance I would die, a five per cent chance my left side would be paralysed and a ten to fifteen per cent chance my arm would be weak for a while but would recover with time (as best I can remember). Thinking the odds sounded pretty good, the operation was scheduled for the following week.

After six hours in theatre, they were still far from finished and would normally have closed up and returned the following day, but my vital signs were very strong, so they continued for a total of ten hours, during which time, Mr Varma never left the operating theatre. Mum was allowed to stay at my bedside for the few days before I came round uttering, "So begins another weary day." – a quote from a Madness song I'd prepared before being anaesthetised. On checking, we discovered my left side was paralysed, and Mr Varma explained that I'd suffered two strokes since the angiogram, making the lesion much deeper than it had originally been and the operation more difficult. I was fairly well-balanced in accepting what happened, knowing there was no way of undoing such things and no point in regret. On the plus side, I was not in the yet-less-fortunate two per cent.

Not being able to exercise limbs I had no control over, I didn't spend much time in physiotherapy. But while in occupational therapy, I remember seeing a patient across the room doing physio. He was learning to run again, still having only limited control over his leg. To my shame, I decided it better to settle for walking as if with a wooden leg than to run like a spastic. Pride is a character flaw that I struggled with for years. Though it doesn't bother me now, when I was younger, I hated looking different.

Three weeks after the surgery, I had my twenty-first birthday party at Rossie with family and a few close friends. Mum tells me I retired to my bed after a short time, still pretty weak. The following year was spent learning to do everything one-handed. Though the leg might seem like the bigger problem, it was actually quite easy to walk, particularly at first with no spasms to contend with, much like walking with a wooden leg.

The thing that annoyed me most about walking in the years to come was, when on a night out with the guys, I'd find myself falling further and further behind as we walked between pubs. This was incredibly frustrating because there was nothing I could do to catch up, and I refused to call on them to wait, for that would make me feel weak.

The greater challenge for now was figuring out how do things one-handed: tying shoelaces, eating meals, cooking, putting a quilt cover on, playing snooker and pool ... the list goes on and on. The only way to really know how hard it is to manage with just one working arm would be to tie one hand behind your back for a few months, any less and you won't come close to feeling the frustration. I adapted surprisingly quickly though, soon tying my own laces, coping with the majority of domestic concerns and even getting pretty good at one-handed snooker.

TEGRETOL

Tegretol is the only anticonvulsant where I'm not exactly sure when the prescription was started or when the dose was raised. But given it is of little consequence, and I cannot bother my doctors with this while in Covid lockdown, my best guess will have to suffice.

Within a few months, I had a grand-mal seizure, meaning the one good thing I thought had come from the operation was not true. The epilepsy was not fixed. The only difference was the head-turning warning was gone; now I just passed out and went into convulsions. A major downer for it ruled out driving, now far more important with the paralysis, so my prescription was changed from Epilim and Phenytoin to 400mg of Tegretol.

Around this time, someone told Mum I should be entitled to disability money, mainly because of the paralysis but also the epilepsy, so I made enquiries and filled out application forms for Disability Living Allowance, where part was for help with mobility and the other for care. The application was rejected, so I contacted our local MP, Ming Campbell, and he provided a letter of support for my claim, but it was again rejected. This had me at a loss, for I knew plenty of people, far less disabled than myself, who were receiving these benefits. Then Mum said a friend told her I should go to Citizens Advice for help as they knew how to fill out the forms.

The eternal optimist, I had been overstating my abilities. For example, if I could manage a task one in every four attempts, I said I could do it, and if I could walk without pain in the early morning though not later in the day, again I said I could. On meeting with the lady at Citizens Advice, she explained that I had to report what I could manage at the worst times not the best, because the assessors would assume I was exaggerating my disabilities in an attempt to get more money. She took me through the questions, filling out the answers for me, and I was awarded low rate for mobility and middle rate for care. Not a huge sum but enough to make a difference.

In the early years after the op, I took up lawn bowling at the Auchtermuchty bowling club, going to the village pretty much every day to play. There was a loner called Jeremy who walked the roads and played bowls. He sold me a great set of bowls, and though usually practising alone, we would occasionally play each other, so I learnt to play precision bowls. Jeremy was a great talent but too reserved to be a champion, and it would seem the same was now true of me. As much as I once loved winning, having developed a fear of losing, I found myself unable to compete in any of the competitions.

When playing for one of the rinks, I was always lead, throwing out the jack and first two bowls. I asked the skip if I could play further down the order, but he said he wanted me at the start, getting us off on the right foot. Eventually growing tired of not participating in the interesting part of the game, I gave up playing for the club and continued alone or with Jeremy. Dad was a great curler, the best around, and I would love to have emulated him at bowls, but having lost the confidence I once had when playing billiards – an effect of brain surgery or the change in medication – there was no chance of that.

On giving up bowls, I switched back to snooker, playing at the Royal Hotel in Auchtermuchty most afternoons. Which brings me to another unfortunate incident.

I was playing with Willie, Tony and a few others. Willie had just chapped me a line of coke on the wooden edge of one of the tables when his girlfriend Shona arrived and, in a fury, scattered the white powder across the room. The next thing I remember I'm sitting in Tony's car getting a lift back to

Rossie. When I asked what happened, he explained that on seeing Shona scatter my coke, I'd punched her.

Let's just say, Shona was a feisty lassie, not the sort to be argued with, never mind punched, and she did not take well to this indiscretion. Fortunately – as I lay on the floor with her punching my head – Tony came to my rescue and pulled her off. My sincere apologies to Shona for being such a bellend – here's hoping she can forgive me. I'd never hit a woman before and never would again … if for no better reason than my own well-being.

Life had become stagnant, so I decided to apply to take an HND in computing at Fife College of Technology in Kirkcaldy. Of course, this meant again using doctor's letters to explain earlier failures. Because the epilepsy still wasn't under control, the Tegretol prescription was increased from 400mg to 800mg, and so I have no real recollection of Kirkcaldy.

After having failed all my first-year exams, I was successful in taking the summer resits but hadn't submitted an HNC project so would have to do that in the second year. I completed second year but didn't sit or pass any HND exams (don't know which) and didn't complete the first-year project, needed for the HNC, so I was left with nothing.

I smoked a fair bit of weed and spent a lot of time at a nightclub called Bentleys, but I have almost no visual memories of this time. Unable to picture any of my friends or even remember their names, it's as if someone has told me what happened, or I've read it in a book, and that is my memory.

Though there for two years, my only clear memory is attending a Raith Rovers football match, having been invited to try the half-price disabled seats. I remember nothing of the game or even who I went with, just a sickening despair on leaving. I hated being treated differently for being disabled and vowed never to return.

On returning from Kirkcaldy, the paper mill had fallen on hard times, and the Major's estate was sold in an attempt to cover losses. I'm not sure, but I think Major Russell had passed away. Moving back to stay with Mum and Dad where they now lived in the burgh of Auchtermuchty, I was placed by Remploy as a temp accounts administrator with Hewlett Packard at South Queensferry.

I didn't like working for Remploy, as at school, the backward children were called remedial, the rems, so the name Remploy, for a company established to help disabled people get work, seemed incredibly demeaning. Who's going to rush off to tell their friends they've got a job in remedial employment. Maybe, in retrospect, an appropriate label for someone stupefied by Tegretol, but nonetheless, the initial placement was only for four months, and hating being thought of as disabled, never mind an idiot, I did not ask for an extension.

Working myself back into Auchtermuchty's social network, I often played pool at the Hollies Hotel with Stuart, Lindsay and Emma. Stuart eventually married Lindsay, but though thinking Emma a really bonny lass, I was far from ready to settle down so never tried to court her. I also played darts for the Hollies with Stuart, Keith and a few others. Our only big win came when playing a team that had already won the league and so decided to try some of our poppers (amyl nitrite) outside the pub. Perhaps the reason we were not very good.

With little else to do with my time, I started hanging out with Jim – a professional layabout – sitting in his flat at Clement Court, getting stoned and playing cards. On one such occasion, having found a load of what he reckoned were opium poppies in an old disused garden across town, we took a couple of plastic bags and headed off to get them, gathering the heads of the plants for boiling in a pot of water, eventually draining the liquid and pouring ourselves a pint each. I remember my first drink tasted all right and felt good. Other than that, I have no more recollection of that day. I woke the following morning at home with my tongue badly bitten, having had a seizure. Not one to be put off by such misadventure, I was back on the path to destruction within a week as Jim had concocted another plan for a hit.

We headed up to the local chemist and got ourselves a bottle of codeine linctus each. On returning to his flat, we kindled up a spliff and drank the cough medicine straight from the bottles, finishing the lot within a matter of minutes. After about an hour of hilarity, we ran out of drink and decided to go to the shop for some beer. I did not recognise anything, road or buildings, as we walked to the shop, and took a seizure on arrival. Jim told me later he'd had no idea what to do so left it to the staff, and a new doctor in Auchtermuchty, Dr Collinson, came to my rescue. Thinking the seizure had paralysed my left side, he got quite a shock and sent me to Ninewells Hospital. Of course there was no new paralysis, but my right arm was badly broken, meaning I could not look after myself, so I was given a stookie and sent to Adamson Hospital in Cupar to be cared for while it healed.

Though the search for utopia through such means ultimately proved fruitless, I did, I'm sure, benefit from the times we spent fishing. The other day, CJ, Stuart's younger brother, reminded me of a trip to Birnie Loch.

Jim had lent me a rod and reel, and it wasn't long before I hooked a large pike. CJ says it almost pulled me into the water – which was extremely deep, being an old quarry – before he grabbed the back of my jacket and held me steady. With the reel handle clenched between my right molars, I wound the line in by circling the rod on the axis of the reel, and after a hectic struggle, we eventually landed the fish. At somewhere between ten and twelve pounds, it was a cracker, worthy of a photo shoot before being returned to the murky depths of the loch.

Soon after, I started working with Fife Council as an accounts administrator. I got the position because I was disabled, and hated that fact almost as much as the work – where my stand-out achievement was to organise a stationery cupboard.

After about a year, a vacancy came up for a trainee accountant. On asking my boss about it, he said I'd need a degree in order to apply. Shocked, I reiterated, "It's a trainee position," but he confirmed a degree was a requirement. So the following week, I took a train down to Herriot Watt University and met with David Marwick, head of first- and second-year computer science. Giving him a full rundown of my academic history and insisting that if he gave me this chance I would not fail again, I must have a gift for exploiting pity, for he agreed to give me a place.

GABAPENTIN

After securing the place at Heriot Watt, my doctor switched my medication from Tegretol – which he said would numb my thinking – to gabapentin, a drug better suited to learning. At first the change was quite emphatic, as if someone had turned a light on. I felt elated and full of confidence, as was clearly demonstrated at David's wedding, where I had the honour to be best man, a role definitely not suited to the likes of me.

The ceremony over, David, CJ and me had a couple of spliffs; so the groom's speech at the reception was a little shorter than expected. Not having made any preparation for my best man's speech, I stood before the crowd … *What should I say?* … I grabbed hold of some Best Wishes cards, from people unable to attend, and started reading them aloud.

Granny Doull shouted, "Can you speak up, Tony? I can hardly hear you."

I countered with, "This is as loud as I speak!"

Then Mum said that I had to toast the bridesmaids, which I understood to be David's duty, but becoming irritated by her nagging, I raised my glass in an off-the-cuff the toast, "Tae a fine set of bridesmaids!"

My finale was to wish Stephen Hendry the best of luck in retaining his world snooker title against Jimmy White, the match having just got underway. This incompetence in public speaking, seemingly down to idiocy, arrogance and laziness, would later take its toll academically.

Leaving the crowd begging for more, I took to the dance floor and spent the majority of the night dancing with my cousin Stella. Thinking her the belle of the ball, I felt no apprehension as she was my cousin, leaving Millrat (one of the groomsmen) a tad pissed off on missing his chance to court her.

Far better than Tegretol, the gabapentin added an extra gear, meaning my memories for the next five years are much clearer, and perhaps more importantly, the initial euphoria on switching from a sedative to a stimulant only lasted a few months.

On receiving the letter of acceptance, I had to get things sorted out with regards to funding, as the Department of Social Security would withdraw my benefits and the student awards agency refused to cover my first year's tuition fees. Anne Trotman, the university's disabled students' advisor, came to the rescue, securing not only funding for fees but also a grant to help with living expenses, which together with a student loan would be ample for the first year.

Moving to the George Burnett Hall of Residence at Riccarton Campus, on the outskirts of Edinburgh, in October 1994, my attitude to learning was completely different, not only going to every class but rewriting notes from the day's lectures into books every night and questioning lecturers on anything not fully understood the following day. I was getting top marks in most subjects, particularly maths and programming, though still mediocre with written projects, things were going well. I really loved my time there, occasionally playing darts with Lee, another "mature" student, and even going out for the odd Coke (now teetotal) with others from our class – though I kept such merriment to an absolute minimum. The only thing that mattered was not failing again, and so, ironically, with working so hard and toeing the line, there's not much to report from these early months.

My classmate, Stuart, a typical ginger Scotsman from Falkirk, noted for his unbound enthusiasm, did say recently that we were well-liked by the dinner ladies, for every Tuesday night, the two of us, often Lee too, would head to the refectory for the half-price special. Always returning for seconds, they would load our plates to the brim, for we were commoners and treated them as equals, whereas some of the other students were a wee bit superior.

A really chilled-out guy called Mark (whose girlfriend, Lisa, was also in our hall) came to me toward the end of the second or third term asking for some help with maths as he'd attended barely any lectures. Having been there myself, I was more than happy to explain two of the three required questions, using examples from past papers. He was very capable and quickly understood, getting an A in the exam the following day.

Mark did get in touch years later on Facebook, and I met with him and Lisa in Edinburgh where they said they were to be married. Most likely alarmed by my erratic manner, they left it at that. Here's hoping all went well for them.

This was the happiest I'd been in years. I wasn't drinking, so there were no comedowns or hangovers, and more importantly, success in work was bolstering my confidence. Then one day, near the beginning of the third term, I had a seizure in Lee's room when playing darts, falling back against a bedside cabinet as I went into convulsions. Waking in my room an hour or so later with searing pains in my back and right side, I dragged myself out of bed and staggered across the campus bent double. Fortunately, it was little more than a hundred meters to the doctors' surgery where I shamelessly begged for their help. Immediately coming to my aid, leaving all else to the side, they gave me morphine to ease the pain and called an ambulance.

I was given more morphine while in the ambulance, so when we arrived at the hospital, the pain had eased considerably. We were met by a young Asian doctor who questioned me, asking what was sore, where it started, how it was now, etc. Then a rather snooty doctor came over to review things. The

Asian doctor suggested we might do a scan of my liver as the pain would seem to be centred on my right side, but the snooty fellow said, "Pay attention to what the patient is saying! Clearly it's appendicitis and that can be easily dealt with tomorrow." Very high on morphine, that sounded fine to me, but as the night went on, the pain got much worse, to a point where a nurse had just given me a shot of morphine and it made no difference. On exclaiming, "It isn't working, the pain is too bad, I can't stay conscious!" I passed out.

When waking the following day, I learnt that the hospital's head surgeon had been called out at 2 a.m. He told me they'd checked the appendix and found nothing so went to the liver where they'd drained about a pint of internal bleeding before cauterising the wound. Had he been half an hour later, my liver would have burst which would have been fatal.

With convalescence scheduled for three weeks, in the hospital, Anne (the disabled students' advisor) brought down lecture notes and coursework from the university each day, and the TV room was left for me to study. The other patients would only come in at 6 p.m. to watch the news, refusing to interrupt my work during the rest of the day. I should add that a young female doctor came round to see me not long after the op, saw my right lung was collapsed, and brought a machine round to reinflate it. I think they put a tube down my throat and pumped air in, but this one's a bit hazy.

I insisted on returning to campus a week early, still quite tired and suffering pain in both my liver and lower back. One of the maths tutors told me not to concern myself further with a tricky question, saying I was clearly exhausted and should settle for an A. Sorry for sounding superior, but I need to make the most of what highlights there were. Passing all my exams that term with three As and a B, winning the Andrew Stewart prize for my tenacity, I had at last successfully completed a year in higher education.

I returned to hospital in the summer to have a further half pint of blood drained from the wound, and thankfully, that was that.

The back pain persisted for several years and was treated with dihydrocodeine ... Sherlock Holmes did his "best thinking" while on opiates, so surely the same should be true for me ...

Second year was a step into a different world. As class rep, I attended monthly meetings with staff, and my work regime remained good. But I stopped rewriting the day's lecture notes each night as I no longer felt that necessary for an academic of my standing. Moving to the new and much more luxurious Robin Smith Hall of Residence, my room had a huge en-suite bathroom with a power shower that ploughed a torrent of water straight onto the floor. It was a double-sized disabled person's room, made especially large so as to accommodate wheelchair access, with a shared kitchen and all the amenities.

There was a girl in our class called Kathy. Other than being blonde, I can't picture her now, but I do remember feeling a strong attraction when we teamed up to do a project together early in second year. As we walked back from the Robin Smith Hall after working on the project, she said she would need some sort of commitment from me, and I told her, "You'd be better off without me as I've always fucked up in the past and would most likely do the same again." Although gabapentin was a far better drug – in that it kept my mind clear and sharp enough to learn – it did nothing to combat the crippling anxiety that came with courting. She said okay, and it was never discussed again.

Stuart recently sent me our class graduation picture, and though I recognise him and Lee, Kathy appears as someone I've never seen before.

On starting the second term of second year, when handed our maths syllabus, I realised it was identical to one from our first year. Effectively, there were two maths classes in first year – one with a higher entry level than the other, but on reaching second year, the classes merged. Inevitably, those who took the lower class would have some catching up to do, and the rest would get an easy time of it for a term. As class rep, looking to impose my new-found authority, I kicked up a stink, refusing to retake the class, and it was suggested I be given an A for attending the exam and answering one question. Thought I'd got one hundred per cent first time round (another highlight), I reluctantly agreed. Again, I'm sorry for being such a prat.

Second year was completed successfully with little else to tell. It is surprising how boring my story becomes when behaving as a "normal academic" would, but fear not, such times were short-lived.

At the outset of third year, Anne Trotman came to me with some "fabulous" news. She'd learnt I was entitled to a back payment of around £8,000 in state benefits for the first two years. But this turned out to be something of a poisoned chalice, for I bought myself a state-of-the-art computer and fell off the wagon. I would get friends to bring cannabis and alcohol up from town, and rarely left my room at Robin Smith other than to get food from the campus shop. Mark, though no longer a student, would often come up to play RAC Rally on the new computer and chill out to music from my prized collection of tapes and CD's.

I did occasionally pop down to class, but the problem with taking all that weed was it made me nervous and very paranoid, to the extent that I was afraid to leave my room in case I met someone I knew. On attending one electrical engineering class, the lecturer asked a question about a circuit he'd drawn on the board. A guy sitting down at the front said the answer was yes, and I instinctively said no, quietly. The lecturer asked him why and he could not explain, then turned to me and asked, "Why not?"

"Because Q1 is not a negative edge."

"Yes, and when will it be?"

"At the next clock pulse."

"Correct."

Kathy was sitting behind me, and I heard her whisper to a friend, "How did he know that?" Then, "He said he'd fuck things up; I don't understand why he's doing this."

In another class, the same guy wrongly answered a question about search algorithms. It was something to do with breaking the pot being searched into several smaller pots, then searching each in turn, and whether that would be faster. He said no, and I said yes. Basically, the average search time was relative to the square of the size of the pot being searched, so reducing the size of the pots, significantly reduces the average search time, even though you will likely have to search more than one pot. When asked why this time, I answered, "Because the search is order n squared." With those being the only classes that I remember attending in the first two terms, correctly answering these two questions gave me an unwarranted confidence in my abilities.

Mid-second term, I sent a hand-drawn Valentine's card to a girl I fancied in Auchtermuchty *(again I cannot picture her face now)*. I spent a fair amount of time creating it while stoned in my room. It was a pencil drawing of a penis smoking a spliff with the caption: Happy Valentine's Day from Puff the Magic Dragon. Thinking it was really funny and sure to make her laugh, instead it frightened her, and I found myself having to write an apology letter promising not to bother her again. This was down to cannabis and dihydrocodeine not the epilepsy drugs. I will not mention her name so as not to cause her further embarrassment.

As we approached the Easter break, I'd completed nothing in the way of classes or coursework for the year so far, and seeing that I was about to blow everything again, I decided I had to get it together. Giving up drinking, weed and smoking, all at once, I put myself through a hellish cold turkey over the third term and summer vacation and somehow managed to catch up with everything and pass my degree exams so qualifying for the honours year. On reflection, quitting cigarettes was a mistake as I started again after the summer, also returning to drink (weekends only) as I now needed a social life, an effect of dihydrocodeine, but I did not return to the cannabis. I know cannabis is loved by many and lauded for its healing qualities, but it never sat well with my epilepsy and definitely made me paranoid.

Somewhere near the start of a hectic honours year, when down town for an evening alone, I met some second-year students in a bar and took them on a pub crawl. At the end of the night (about 1 a.m.) while waiting alone for a taxi back to Riccarton, three gorgeous girls wearing short, red dresses asked if I'd like to share a cab. We chatted on the way, and on arriving at the campus, they asked if I fancied a *coffee* as they all felt like one. Overcome by the relentless anxiety that crippled me whenever I was courted by beautiful women, I said, "Sorry, no, I have an early class."

This was my biggest downer yet, and feeling pathetic, I decided I had to do something about it. A friend once told me he had access to prostitutes, so I asked him for the number. Calling the next day, I asked for two girls, as three was beyond my means. They arrived that afternoon, one in her mid-thirties and the other about my age. The older one stripped naked, undressed me and did a lap dance with us both naked before putting a condom on me. Then the second girl, saying it was her first time working, jumped on top and did her thing. I won't go into more detail as I'm sure you're not at all interested, but let's just say my frustrations were relieved for a good while thereafter. I wrote two cheques for £150, and they left.

I was reminded of this not long ago, as Stuart, who also came to live at Robin Smith in fourth year, had seen or heard there was a black limo parked outside the hall for about an hour with a driver/pimp sitting waiting. It would seem all at the hall were aware of my indulgence, not that I cared.

About this time, I met a business school student called Didier. He was a true gentleman, a black man from Burundi. I thought he might be aristocracy but never asked, thinking that would be uncouth, and more importantly, I didn't care. There was many a time he'd foot the bill for our taxi back to campus when the rest of us had empty pockets after a night on the town.

One night, before going into town, Didier and me went to a bar in Currie. While we waited for our drinks, a local came over and said, "Students have no idea about the real world; they cannae handle themselves against real men." As Didier turned toward him, he stepped back saying, "I can see that you would be a good fighter, coming from Africa, but him, no"—looking at me—"he's just a spoilt little rich boy."

As I stood up, Didier put his hand on my chest and said, "No, he's just trying to wind you up. Ignore him; he's not worth bothering about." And so I did, and we headed off to the town.

Later that night, when en route to the East End Subway, my left ankle went over on a cobble stone. It was so painful I thought it broken and took a taxi back to campus. On hobbling down to the doctors' surgery the following morning, an X-ray revealed it wasn't broken, just badly swollen with a torn tendon. Far better had it been broken as the tendon ached for nigh on a year, even with dihydrocodeine.

About half an hour after recording this memory, when walking in the woods, my left ankle felt swollen and started to ache in the same way it had back then. It only lasted about an hour, but what a bizarre way to step back in time.

Time for another "failed romance", and this may sound like an opiate fantasy, a concoction of my mind linking what were in fact unrelated events, but it's what I believed at the time so it should be mentioned. We were sitting in the student union one afternoon having a beer, with three hot girls sitting at the other side of the room. One was sitting across a bench seat with her legs up perpendicular to us, wearing nothing other than a pair of tights from the waist down. Her friend said, "What are you doing? He can see your vagina."

"No, he can't," she replied, "I'm side-on to him."

I should point out that me and my two friends were the only other people in the room, and my friends were paying no heed to her. Our taxi arrived a few minutes later, and we were off.

A week later, back in the union, a gorgeous girl dressed up to the nines stood alone at the bar. After a while, I got up to order drinks. I said nothing to her as the usual anxiety was burning, paid for the round and returned to my seat. A couple of minutes later, she went storming out with a face like thunder. As she passed, I noticed her legs and realised it was the same girl.

The following day while waiting in the shop, I heard a girl say to her friend, "He must have known; someone must have told him," while looking at me. At the time, I wasn't sure what she meant. Then later that day as I sat alone in the refectory having lunch, a very handsome guy across the room was looking at me with weird, gazing eyes. Watching for a bit before turning back to my food, I heard him say, "Nope, definitely not." His friend replied, "He *must* be gay!" – but he insisted not.

Finally connecting the dots but still "painfully shy" (as I once overheard myself described by another girl I fancied), I decided to leave it at that. Whatever the truth, it was just another example of my inability to connect with women.

Studying went well as we tended to only go out on weekends, and the rest of the week was devoted to work. On one such weekend when on a binge session – to be honest I'm not sure who was all there – we were sitting in the West End Subway nightclub when Stuart asked if I wanted another pint.

I said, "No, get me a nip instead."

And a wee while later, he arrived back with a pint and a nip. I looked at him despairingly, "I told you, I don't want a pint!"

"Stop being a baby and get it down you!" he insisted, so I picked up the pint glass and threw its contents at Stuart.

Next thing I know, there's a guy standing in front of us shouting and roaring something. The bouncer speaks to him, comes over, takes me by the scruff of the neck and throws me out. Angry because the bouncer would not explain why, I waited in the street for the guy to come out. About an hour later, as the club was closing up for the night, he walked through the door and stopped in front of me, I took note of exactly where his head was, looked up to the sky and punched him hard in the face before looking down again. He fell to the ground but soon recovered, got to his feet and knocked me over. I was lying on my back, with him punching the side of my head as I pulled him toward me by his T-shirt, hoping to land a headbutt – fighting is a whole different kettle of fish with a paralysed side. I felt his shirt tearing as the bouncers pulled him off.

Looking back as he walked down the road, he shouted, "It's not over!"

I smiled and touched my cheek to remind him of the three knuckle marks now clearly showing on his face.

This seemed a fair outcome until Stuart told me what actually happened. Apparently, when I threw the beer at Stuart, he saw it coming and ducked to the side, and it went all over the guy I ended up fighting with. So once again, I find myself offering a sincere apology, though this time to someone I don't know and will likely never see again.

I haven't said much about gabapentin and its side effects for they were relatively trivial. Though in itself, only a moderate neural stimulant – in combination with the dihydrocodeine I'd been taking for back pain since being hospitalised in first year, I was definitely not myself.

Another example would be the time we went into town and one of the bouncers at a night club refused to let me in, saying I'd had too much. When the guys came back out, on realising I'd been refused entry, I told them that I'd smashed the windscreen of what I knew to be the bouncer's car in a nearby side street. They would not believe that I'd smashed the windscreen, which of course I had not, so I punched my fist through the window in the driver's door, thinking that this would demonstrate my sincerity. Cutting my hand pretty badly, we wrapped it in a T-shirt or something of the like, and eventually, after a couple of refusals, found a taxi that would give me a lift back to campus.

I was walking through the main building at Riccarton, with the white cloth on my hand, now soaked in blood, when I saw a security guard running toward me from the far end of the corridor that led to reception. As he drew near, he got his radio from his pocket and said, "It's all right; it's just Tony," then kindly took me up to their station at the main entrance and bandaged my hand. So though this drug combo did not seem to impede learning or memory, it was far from ideal.

It's hard to justify behaviour like this, but in these early years I was only ever aggressive when taking dihydrocodeine or coke. I've only taken coke three times in my life, and the highs were much like that of dihydrocodeine, particularly when taken with alcohol.

A year or so later, I learnt that drugs like dihydrocodeine are highly addictive, and the brain will actually mimic pain in order to get more, so I decided to stop taking it for a trial period. After about two months, the pain in my back was completely gone, and more importantly, my behaviour considerably calmed.

Somehow managing to survive these escapades, I had a good honours year, spending a great deal of time working on my dissertation developing an algorithm that would establish the direction of the primary source of light for a digital image. Basically, creating a database of image patterns, where the light source was known, using a data structure to store the intensity variances in blocks of sixteen pixels together with the direction of the light. The images were also scaled down so they could be analysed less intricately, where the final scaled image was just one block of sixteen pixels. In the end, the algorithm was relatively successful but very slow, as it took a huge amount of time to search the database for a best match.

You may have noted I don't make much mention of epilepsy, and that is because I don't want to dwell on banal recurrences of the same old thing. During my time at Herriot Watt, I would have had a seizure every two to three months, but there are two that have to be recorded.

We had four honours exams. Two were fine, but on the evening before one of the finals, I had a seizure and, as a consequence, fell asleep in the exam. Then another seizure on the morning of the last, and I didn't show up at all. Normally, this would result in automatic failure, because there are no resits for honours, but this was brought to appeal by my good friend and mentor, Dr Manuel Trucco, and so I had to attend an appeals tribunal. On being asked about the exam I fell asleep in, I said my mind had gone blank, and though one question was an exact match to my course project, it had made no sense at the time. The doctor was able to confirm the seizure on the morning of the final exam as I went down to the surgery on waking so they could see the tearing on my tongue.

On going to learn my fate from Manuel a few days later, he told me I'd just got an ordinary. Then laughed, saying, "No, don't be silly, it's a 2.2."

Though I knew this was a fair grade, given the circumstances, I was still disappointed.

The following day, Anne Trotman emailed me to see if I'd be interested in an MPhil scholarship. I went straight to Manuel and asked if he would be my supervisor, and he readily agreed. So things were beginning to look up. I brought my family to graduation – a day they most likely thought would never come – won the Andrew Stewart prize again, which helped in easing my disappointment at not scoring a higher degree, and meant I had my picture taken with Lord Mackay.

After a photo shoot with friends and family; me, Stuart, Lee and some others headed to town to get pissed for the first time as graduates. Stuart bought himself a nip of single malt from the Haymarket bar and offered me a sip. On learning he'd paid £50, I declined, insisting he have it himself. *On reflection, a mistake as I'm teetotal now and so will never have the chance again.*

I met Boutros early in my master's year. A huge black guy from central Africa, he was a warden at the Robin Smith Hall of Residence. We first met the day after I came back from the pub in a stupor, put the chip pan on and went to bed, only to find the kitchen full of black reek on getting up the next morning. The fire alarm hadn't gone off because the kitchen sensor was heat sensitive, but on closing the door and opening the window, there was enough breeze to blow smoke under the door and into the hallway setting off the smoke sensor there, and not long after, Boutros arrived with four fire engines.

It was either then or in a games room where I challenged him to a game of table tennis. A girlfriend of his looked surprised, saying, "Boutros is very good."

But like a gentleman, he agreed to play. When we reached 11–10 to him, he said, "Cheers, great game," and I said, "No, it's first to twenty-one." So we continued. When it reached 21–20, he claimed victory again, and I said, "No, you have to win by two clear points," at which he seemed a tad frustrated, but we carried on, with him eventually winning 27–25.

We became good friends during my master's year, occasionally drinking in town with Didier and some others. I remember one time in particular, Boutros told me a guy was trying to get in with a girl he'd just broken up with, right in front of him, showing no respect. He wasn't sure about the culture here in Scotland but wanted to sort things out – so asked if I thought that would be acceptable. I told him to do whatever he felt necessary but to make sure he had a quick exit ready should anything go wrong. A couple of days later, I heard he went back to the club and taught the bounder a valuable lesson before leaving by a back door, escorted by a friendly bouncer. I'm not sure I was the best one to come to for advice, but all's well that ends well.

I joined Manuel's lab group, taking on a project to recognise features in sequential video images so as to stitch them together using a geometric transform, creating a mosaic – in a similar but less elaborate way to how Google Earth was later created. Initially, I used my dissertation code to find the features, and having tracked their movement between frames, stitched them together using an affine transform. I got positive results fairly quickly, though the feature tracking was very slow because of the complexity of my search algorithm.

There was another fellow in the lab, who was also working on this problem, funded by a French research company. He'd been working on it for some time and still had no positive results, so his funding was withdrawn. And when he left, Manuel was able to get that funding transferred to me.

Manuel suggested I try using a feature tracker that Stratus (a PhD fellow) had coded, and rather than the affine, we switched to a slightly more effective perspective transform. The revised algorithm was highly effective for its time, both in speed and quality of imagery.

Then, with things apparently going so well, I was asked to give a presentation of my work to our lab group. And this is where it all fell flat. Though I worried obsessively about girls, it would seem that was the only part of my brain's worrying mechanism that worked. On top of that gabapentin did have one adverse side effect – it made me think I was a genius. The combination of thinking I was a genius, and not worrying, so not bothering to review, refine, or scrutinise my writing – believing all would listen in awe – was to prove catastrophic. I overheard one of the girls say, "How can he be so brilliant a programmer and such a terrible speaker?" She'd said, "brilliant programmer," and that was all that mattered to me; but it turns out presentation is paramount in academic circles, and so, soon after, I was instructed by the company who'd switched funding to me to cease work on the project and not publish my findings.

Leaving me with no option but to write up my thesis in the hope it might suffice for an MPhil. This meant it would officially be published as it would go into the university library but would not be published elsewhere. When taking on to write up the work, I was far from confident – now aware I was no genius – and written English had always been my Achilles heel. But I trudged along, using plenty of images to fill the pages, and things seemed to be going well.

Then one morning on arriving at the lab, I heard whispering among the others, and when I checked my email, I realised why. Manuel had sent an email to my external examiner at Edinburgh University, explaining that my writing skills were pretty weak, but I was an excellent programmer and problem-solver (or words to that effect), and asking him to keep that in mind. Unfortunately, he'd inadvertently sent a copy to all in the lab, including me. Manuel came rushing to apologise, insisting he hadn't intended to send it to anyone other than the external examiner. Of course, I accepted his apology, knowing he hadn't said anything that wasn't entirely true. It's a bit like music – I know I have a terrible voice, having heard recordings, but I still sing because it sounds good in my head.

It was around this time I went up to Shetland for my cousin Leslie's wedding and met Marie-Anne for the first time. She was a really beautiful Norwegian girl, *sadly, again I cannot remember her face*, but we hit it off from the start. On returning to the mainland, I completed my thesis and was able to defend it at viva with only a couple of minor changes suggested. One of the girls in the lab told me I was the first in Scotland to get an MPhil in just one year, and though I knew another guy in electrical engineering had been trying for the same, but he'd had to continue for another year, I'm pretty sure she was just saying that to cheer me up. On completion, Manuel did say I'd done a great job of writing up, and he would certainly give it to future students to read. Though I would not get a PhD, I was happy enough and ready to move on.

I continued working in the lab for a few months, moving to Lothian Road to share a flat with Boutros and three others. First to see the place, Boutros and me had the pick of the rooms. When we asked if the smaller rooms were cheaper, the landlord insisted they were all £500, so we took the biggest two, only to learn later that the other three were let out for considerably less.

I was getting very fond of Marie-Anne, often calling Norway and chatting long into the night. I eventually persuaded her to come and see Edinburgh, with the hope I might convince her to come live with me in Scotland. Though I was a little nervous, she quickly had me won me over with her relaxed Scandinavian approach to sexuality. It was a fantastic week, and after she left, though we kept in touch by telephone, I found myself longing for her company. So, I went over to Norway to meet her son and check things out, before coming back and packing my bags, saying my reluctant farewells to Manuel and the gang at Herriot Watt, and heading across the North Sea to live in Norway.

Arriving with clothes, a few tattered books and academic stuff including data drives and software. I had lots of fun with Marie-Anne but found the Norwegian tongue impossible to learn. I spent many hours trying to get a grasp of the language but fared even worse than I had with French and English at school. An indication that the part of my brain devoted to language had been impaired by the vascular malformation and was further diminished after surgery. I did apply for one job in Oslo and attended an interview to work as a website designer, but I had no interest in such things as would have been obvious to those interviewing me. They did get back in touch, inviting me to come for a second interview, but I left it at that.

Marie-Anne's son went to stay with his father every second weekend, and though well behaved and settled in the second week with us, on returning from his father's he was an absolute nightmare for several days before calming down again. I've never had any interest in children, and though we'd likely have been fine without the visits to his father, I was not prepared to have my life so adversely affected by another man.

I decided the only hope was to find work outside Norway, and have Marie-Anne join me later. But as we drove to the airport, only six weeks after my arrival, she said she would not leave Norway as she could not split her son from his father, admitting she'd only suggested otherwise because she believed I would want to stay.

On arriving back in Scotland, I went to Herriot Watt to see if they could help with finding work in the UK, and they pointed me to a position as a research scientist with the Ministry of Defence. I did, by chance, meet Boutros that day, and he told me to stay well away from Lothian Road as the landlord was absolutely fuming. Apparently, I left him with a telephone bill of almost a thousand pounds – with the calls to Norway – and he said he'd have me blacklisted so I'd never get a flat to rent in Edinburgh again. I laughed, saying that'll teach him to lie about the price of the rooms. My interview with the MOD was successful, and I would start working at their Bincleaves site in Weymouth a few months later, once my security clearance was completed.

I decided to stop off and see Aunt Daphne, Uncle Monty and my cousins, Gary and Chris, en route to Weymouth. Gary took it on himself to introduce me to the Southsea night life. On one such occasion, we ended up in a nightclub down by the front. Already having had a fair few drinks, Gary went straight to the bar and ordered six bottles of Bacardi Breezer. We sat at a table upstairs, looking down on the dance floor, and after a while, Gary asked me about picking up girls. He said he always got nervous and could I give him some advice. Remember we were both pissed, so I said, "Of course, just go up to them, say hello, and if they seem enthusiastic, chat about whatever you think they might be interested in."

There were two fairly hot girls standing at the bar behind me, so Gary said, "Right I'm going for it," and headed to the bar. I remained at the table, looking the other way, my eyes glazed, as the Bacardi wrenched at my gut.

A few minutes later, Gary – who is six foot five, by the way – drifted past, cradled by the armpits, as two very large bouncers marched him toward the exit.

As they passed, he shouted, "You can't throw me out, my cousin's a cripple!" while pointing at me, but they continued to take him on his way, and I burst out laughing so bad I almost threw up. This might surely be taken as a clear indication not to come to me for advice on matters of the heart.

CLONAZEPAM

Before leaving Southsea, I met with a doctor my aunt knew. Apparently, she'd found this great new epilepsy medication that would help me relax with almost no side effects. I do now remember her reading from a book on side effects and saying it might cause mental issues. But she light-heartedly dismissed this and admitted that she had no idea what "mental issues" meant, then assured me that the patients she was prescribing it to had suffered no adverse effects. Switching to clonazepam (1mg daily) felt quite wonderful *(hardly surprising given I now know that 1mg of clonazepam is equivalent to 10mg of Valium)*. All my anxiety disappeared, and I headed off to Weymouth with the wind in my sails.

On arriving in Weymouth, I rented a flat from a relation of one of the guys at the Portland site. Bincleaves set me up in my own office with a new superfast computer, but I can't tell you much about the work, having signed the Official Secrets Act.

Though taking on some interesting assignments, I struggled to maintain concentration, and reading was becoming ever more difficult in that I would have to go over the text time and time again, and even then, I could barely make sense of it. When asked to present my work at an MOD conference, I was so nervous I passed it to one of my colleagues to present on my behalf. I must have seemed quite an extraordinary character to those working around me.

Within a couple of months of switching to clonazepam I started to have tremors/spasms down my paralysed left side, making walking very difficult. Alcohol was the only thing that seemed to help, so I spent all of my free time in the pubs drinking and playing one-handed pool. Once, when temporarily relocated to Malvern, I beat Britain's number five professional pool player. To be fair to him, he had come to a local pub to do an exhibition where he played the regulars, and on letting me break, I cleared up without him getting a shot.

My first bad chest infection started while I was in Malvern, forcing me to return to Weymouth and take some time off. On seeing a doctor, I was issued with blue and brown inhalers which I continued to use while on clonazepam. *It turned out that the chest infections – twice every year – and always being short of breath, were an allergic reaction to the drug, but that wasn't realised until many years later.*

Both Chris and Gary stopped by for a night out in Weymouth, but where Chris' visit just involved meeting with him and one of his pals from the army, having a few drinks and a good laugh, Gary's was more of an adventure. We had a night going round the pubs in town, playing pool and getting ever more pissed, before eventually arriving back at my local. As we stood having a cigarette outside, just before last orders, Gary started shouting at two guys across the square. I have no idea why, but he called them a couple of tossers. At this, one ran after Gary, punching me in the left eye as he went past.

I woke the following morning in hospital to find a message saying Gary had been arrested, along with the number for the police station. I hired a taxi to pick him up and take him to my flat for his stuff, as he had to rush back to work in Southsea. Later on that day, the guys in the pub explained that, after punching me, the fighter went after Gary. He was punching Gary's head while holding him up against a wall before a couple of my mates pulled him off and held on to him until the police arrived. The police handcuffed the fighter and pushed him into a panda car. Then, on seeing me lying unconscious on the pavement, Gary ran across and started kicking the car while shouting at the guy inside, and was, needless to say, arrested himself.

A few days later, the police contacted me to see if I wanted charges brought, but given it was Gary who had stirred up the trouble, I decided to leave it at that. Gary was charged with destruction of police property or something of the like, and I still have floaters in my left eye to this day, perhaps poetic justice for that poor lad at the Edinburgh nightclub.

While I was in the south, Chris got married, and my behaviour at his wedding was subtly different to that at my brother's. Able to take a clonazepam just before things got underway, I was very calm and relaxed at the outset, reeling off a string of jokes learnt in the Weymouth pubs. The biggest laugh came during the meal when I demonstrated how to clear nose hairs using a lighter. The flint wasn't working properly, and by the time it eventually sparked, my nose had filled with gas. I breathed out immediately on seeing the flame, with plumes of fire shooting from both nostrils, like that of a dragon. There was no dancing this time round, and as the night passed, I became more and more agitated. The pros and cons of clonazepam were already beginning to tell.

I worked at Bincleaves for eighteen months, before leaving to take on a PhD scholarship at the University of New Hampshire in the United States. Still receiving group emails from the gang at Herriot Watt, I had learnt about the chance in America and secured the scholarship based on my work in Edinburgh. I can't remember the names of any of my colleagues in Weymouth, but I do remember my immediate boss saying he thought my leaving was a mistake. At the time, I imagined he didn't want to lose me and my work, having become inexplicably sure of my abilities despite having made little real progress, but with hindsight, I'm sure he could see I wouldn't manage a PhD.

As regards epilepsy, I had a good few fits while in Weymouth. Twice waking in hospital after being picked up by ambulance, having had a seizure while out on the town.

Otherwise just waking at home in the morning, feeling very tired with a badly bitten tongue. So clonazepam was of no value in controlling seizures, though it did seem to ease anxiety.

Having taken a tablet before going to work, I would feel great for the first few hours of the day, but at around lunchtime, I'd start to feel a bit edgy, and as the afternoon passed, I became progressively more agitated. On arriving back at my flat after work, I'd take the second tablet of the day and feel great again, so I'd head off out to the pub. Though hating the anxiety/calm rollercoaster, I made no attempt to get the medication changed – as that must surely be better than being anxious all the time.

Of course I was wrong; there would have been far less anxiety in the down time were it not for the huge swing the other way after taking a pill. It's like the ripples on throwing a stone into a pool of water; initially the crest of a wave forms where the stone hit the water, but a trough will soon follow. Where with no stone, the pool remains flat.

I sold the stuff from my flat and headed to America to take the PhD in offshore engineering, sharing a beautiful cabin/house in Durham with an undergrad called Jake and a French guy called Emanuel. Not long after getting settled in, I was given a task to clean up some sonar data files. It was a fairly straightforward removal of unneeded data from each record in the files. The job was done within a few hours, and one of the senior lab members called me a real pro. Incredibly, that is the only academic work I remember doing in my eight months at UNH.

So, what happened in America? On my first day there, our very sexy departmental secretary took me to Portsmouth in her soft-top car to see student residences. It was a fantastic day, and as we drove with the roof folded down, her skirt was blowing up in the wind so I could see her panties, Marilyn

Monroe style. She took me to see the student flat she was sharing with some other girls. No one was in, and when she showed me her bed, I remember wishing I had the nerve to ask if she fancied a *coffee*.

On my first visit to what would become my local – Libby's Bar and Grill – while sitting on a stool at the bar, some girls came in for a drink, and as they went over to sit at a table, one of them said, "No, he's faking it." Not sure what they meant, I asked the barman, and he told me it was my Scottish accent. Shortly after, Jake arrived. When I told him they thought my accent was fake, he went over and told them I really was from Scotland. They invited us to join them in a game of pool, saying they were up on a day trip from Boston and would soon have to head off for their bus. But before leaving, one of the girls invited me outside to share a line of coke.

Later that evening, one of the barmen challenged me to a game of pool for twenty dollars. I never turned down a chance to show off my talents at one-handed pool, so he broke off, and I cleared up without him getting another shot. He seemed a bit stunned, so I offered double or quits, and he agreed, but said I should break this time. Asking if he was sure, he insisted, so I broke and cleared up with one shot. Pretty annoyed, he paid up but refused to play anymore, declaring me a hustler. I've rarely taken coke, but Alex Higgins won the world snooker title while high on coke, so you can be fairly sure that's why I played so well that day. We spent the rest of the night drinking, putting songs on the jukebox and playing pool. I liked Durham.

It wasn't long before I had a seizure and was taken to hospital where they gave me a full-body MRI – *which I could not afford and, not having health insurance, did not pay for as it was done without my consent.* When I woke, still hazy after the seizure, a doctor asked me why there was a metal plate at the back/top of my skull. I said I wasn't sure, but I'd had brain surgery in 1988. Then he asked when I'd broken my back, I said never, and he showed me an image with a crack through the third vertebrae up. He assured me it had been broken, perhaps some years ago, but it was now completely healed. Thinking back, the only time it could have happened would be when my liver almost burst after the seizure at Herriot Watt. No wonder my back ached for so long after the operation.

Recently, on being referred for an MRI of my pancreas, I was told there were "multiple surgical staples and clips along the margins of the post-surgical cavity in the right frontal and temporal lobes" – left in my head after the brain surgery. Meaning I can't have an MRI now as these staples and clips are ferromagnetic. Of course, I can't be sure, but I believe the MRI in America is why I don't recognise Kathy in our Heriot Watt graduation picture, cannot visualise Marie-Anne and have no memory of the work I did at UNH other than that first week.

Two days after being reminded about the surgical clips, I began to feel [remember] pains in my head. Not a headache as such but sharp localised pains in the front (above my eyes) and back of my skull – the same pains I felt for several weeks after the MRI (I can't be sure for how long). At the time, I thought it was down to the seizure, but I hadn't felt pain like that since the brain surgery. As earlier with the ankle, it was a weird step back in time that only lasted for a few hours. A good thing, for I did not realise we can remember pain by experiencing it as actual pain.

I decided to have a CT brain scan done for comparison with the one from 1994, as was referenced in my medical records identifying the surgical staples and clips, because some five years after the MRI in 2002, I remember finding a metal clip of sorts tangled in the hair on the back of my neck, next to a bleeding boil, and thinking it might be a surgical clip that had been pulled through my brain by the MRI, with it only now making its way to the surface. On having the scan, I was told there are "multiple surgical staples and clips", but the 1994 CT scan has been lost, so we cannot make a direct comparison (£430 down the drain).

I'm a little unsure of these memories, as I was heavily sedated on 1.5mg clonazepam daily when finding the "surgical clip". Though the memories do feel real, the implications can never be proven, perhaps rendering their inclusion here redundant. But as much as I hate conjecture like this, my objective is to record all key memories, so it has to be mentioned.

I quickly learnt to tip well, because in the States you don't pay for your drinks as you get them, rather you build up a tab and pay it off at the end of the night. I usually had a dark-haired waitress with sparkling eyes looking after me, so tipping her thirty to forty per cent meant I always got a very good measure. One evening, rather than waitressing, she was tending the bar downstairs, so I went down to play pool. Drinking whiskey and ginger ale, in a tall glass, with very generous measures, after a while I started to feel dizzy, and staggering around, I eventually fell to the floor. Of course I had to leave.

While walking back to the cabin, I was picked up by the local police for walking unsteadily. They tied my hands behind my back using one of those plastic cable ties, which was bloody sore on my left wrist. I tried to explain that I was disabled, but they paid no heed, pushed me into the back of the car and took me to Portsmouth for a night in the cells. Having a hellish sore head when released the next day, I took a taxi back home and went straight to bed to sleep it off. The waitress concerned was not allowed to work the downstairs bar again, not because I'd complained, but rather, Libby had somehow got wind of what happened. Given that I was a heavy drinker, and this had never happened before or since, I'm sure my incoordination that night was, at least in part, down to the MRI.

Toward the end of summer, we had a party at our place with lots of booze and all that jazz. Standing chatting to a girl on the top of five wooden steps that led to our front door, I lost my footing and toppled forward. Holding my right arm to my side in a drunken combat roll to break the impact on landing, I continued as if in one fluid movement, back to my feet, lifted my bottle of beer and proclaimed, "I didn't spill a drop." Quite an achievement for someone with a paralysed side. I think it was at this same party that Emanuel and me had something of an altercation. Though I'd liked Jake from the outset, Emanuel was another kettle of fish, maybe because his French arrogance clashed with my own. As best as I can recall, he was running around showing off in front of the girls when he started taunting me, saying I wouldn't dare hit him with the empty two litre plastic bottle in my hand. This was a grave mistake as my brother will testify.

While at a New Year's Eve party in David's garden, I lifted one of those trigger spray bottles and threatened to spray him. He leant forward with his eyes wide open, right in my face, saying, "You can't squirt that at me because it has weedkiller in it, neh neh!" I immediately pulled the trigger, and he had to run off and wash his eyes out (sorry, bro).

So, you can be sure I whacked Emanuel hard on the forehead with the empty plastic bottle. After reeling back in shock, he lunged toward me, but Jake and some others grabbed hold of him until he calmed down. To be fair, though there was loud bang, he was not hurt at all.

A few days later, one of Emanuel's gorgeous classmates came into the cabin while we were sitting watching telly. Undoing her coat to reveal she was wearing nothing other than a white see-through teddy, she looked at Emanuel and said, "Are you free?"

He jumped up, saying, "Yes, follow me," and left for his room.

She walked up to me, teasing her fingers over her silk-covered, clean-shaven crotch, "I keep my vagina nice, if you're ever interested …" then followed Emanuel to his bed.

Man, was I jealous of him that day. But bringing this vision for me to ponder helped greatly in easing tensions there on in.

Late in October, I realised there was no money going into my bank account, and on asking my supervisor why, he told me I was only paid in the summer months. My scholarship would cover my fees during the terms, but I would not get a wage. So, I should have been saving my money rather than blowing it in the pub. Due to it being an honest mistake on my part, he was able to get money from a charitable fund, effectively meaning I got a double wage for the summer.

I have a vague recollection of going to Jake's parents' place for Thanksgiving. It was a beautiful rural home somewhere in New England. His father carved up the turkey while explaining that the dark meat makes you sleepy, and I enjoyed a huge feast followed by some very hazy images of autumn colours viewed through aching eyes as we drove home the following day.

Because seizures are so traumatic on the brain, I have very little recollection of any, even post-seizure, so it was several hours after first writing about this trip before I remembered having had a fit. An unexpected reminder of how lucky I am now.

I'm not sure of the timing for this next outing, not that it really matters. Jake had somehow got the use of an old station wagon, so we decided to party in Portsmouth. Arriving at a bar that was masquerading as an old English pub, we decided to try their Gaelic Warriors – a cocktail: one-third Guinness, one-third cider, and one-third Jameson's whiskey, served in a pint glass. Needless to say, there was much merriment. After a while, we headed out to a country cottage rented by another group of students. To be honest, I don't have much recollection of what happened there, but on leaving, we were driving slowly down a narrow road when Jake decided to stop and check with the car behind to see if they knew where we were. On stopping, there was a considerable bang as the car behind ran into the back of ours. No serious damage was done, though there were a couple of girls crying in the back seat of our car – fortunately, from nothing more than shock. As we continued, a police car passed us going the other way, and Jake immediately turned off the road and parked up in a driveway, for apparently in America, at that time, you could not be charged with drunken driving unless stopped on a main road. Sadly, I can't remember exactly what happened next, but I suspect we just carried on home after sitting a while, for I don't recall any trouble with the police.

On a lighter note, I do remember getting caught out in torrential rain while walking back home from the lab. I ran as best I could toward the shelter of a small railway bridge but was completely soaked within seconds. Fortunately, a kind gentleman gave me a lift back to the house. On another day, soon after, the weather was so hot – around 40°C – the air conditioning failed at the university, and everyone went to Libby's Bar and Grill, it being the only place in town with working air-con. At the opposite extreme, in winter when it reached minus 40°C, I fell in the snow when getting out of Ford's car and had to hold my hand under the cold tap to prevent ice-burn. A few days later, I woke in the morning to find the place so cold that the cup of tea on my bedside cabinet was frozen solid. After dressing under the quilt, I hurried to the living room to find the heating off, the outside boiler having burst. We ended up burning books in a desperate attempt to get a fire lit.

It was around this time a brown bear started raking through our bins for scraps – that being one of my most prized memories.

I should return to Ford, the Good Samaritan who gave me a lift the night I fell in the snow. He was a big guy with red hair and a red beard. As one of the bouncers at Libby's, he often gave me a lift home at the end of the night, once even taking me for a joyride down Route 1 on the back of his Harley Davidson – an awesome experience. Occasionally spending an afternoon at his place, we'd sit toking weed and listening to Pink Floyd – he had every album they'd ever released. Ford told me he was a felon, though as best I can recall, he never actually said what he'd done. He struck me as the sort who thought the Hell's Angels a bunch of pussies. Indeed, I think he said exactly that. A good-hearted fellow, knowing we were a bit strapped for cash, he'd come round with his snow plough and clear our driveway at no charge in the winter. He did later come visit me in Scotland, but sadly, I have almost no recollection of that time.

Out of money again by spring, I told my supervisor there was no point in me continuing with my studies as – because I was disabled – I would not be allowed to take part in the upcoming summer expedition to map the floor of a nearby lake. There was no point me becoming an offshore engineer if I could not go offshore. I got some more money from the charitable fund, or Mum and Dad (I'm not sure which), to pay for my flight home, and that pretty much sums up my time at UNH.

Though achieving absolutely nothing academically, I did return home with some amazing memories. If I make any money from telling this story, I will do my utmost to repay my debt to the charity that saved my ass. Never having been made to feel more welcome, I'm still a little downhearted at not making more of my American adventure.

On returning to live with Mum and Dad in Auchtermuchty, I continued to look for work, but it was becoming ever more difficult to explain my past. I applied for a good number of jobs, mainly in England, and was invited to attend an interview for one where I'd be developing software to stitch together video sequences into a 3D mosaic. The sort that's now used to sell houses, where potential buyers can take a virtual walk through a property online.

I was very unsure of myself. When asked, "What unusual thing should be taken into account when processing an image in Fortran?" – Fortran being the computer language they would be programming in – I was at a complete loss. After prompting with several hints, the interviewer eventually gave up and told me the image must be transposed because of the way Fortran stores data. I did remember when it was explained to me, but my mind was a mush. Whereas most people become more able as their careers progress, the opposite was true for me.

Though offering to work for free until I'd proven my worth, I did not get the job, instead, they politely apologised and said that would not be feasible. I was back at square one. In the year to come, there was drinking, getting stoned and playing pool in Auchtermuchty while continuing to apply for jobs, but there were no more interviews.

Back when doing the short stint at Hewlett Packard (accounts), my boss had asked if I'd like to create a spreadsheet, and I'd shied away, saying I'd never done one before. Now Mum and Dad asked me to manage the accounts for their taxi business, and with great enthusiasm, I got stuck in, building a spreadsheet to record all monetary transactions. It wasn't that complicated, just enough to calculate VAT, and my reckoning was passed to an accountant anyway.

On the plus side, I was able to create a spreadsheet, suggesting clonazepam was not as debilitating as Tegretol.

But staying focused while inputting the numbers proved exhausting, so I dreaded the work. I continued doing their quarterly returns for a good many years until Mum and Dad eventually retired. *The distress that came from being robbed of my intellect might best be compared to that of a priest losing his soul.*

I'd better make some mention of exploits with cousins, Andy and Dale, else I might never here the end of it. The one that comes to mind, around this time, was a night when we'd gone on the bevy to Perth. We were tossed out of Wetherspoon's earlier than planned when Andy and me knocked over a table of drinks while arm-wrestling. Nevertheless, I'd had a load of vodka & Red Bull, so not long after arriving at the Ice Factory night club, I had to pee. Leaving the others at the main bar, I found myself at the end of a maze of corridors with no sign of any toilets. About to wet myself, I peed in a corner, thinking there was no one around, but of course, one of the bouncers came past and threw me out. They told me to go home, but not having enough money to pay for a taxi, I told them I'd have to wait until my friends came out. And so the police arrived, and I was locked up for the night.

I'm beginning to wish I could cut some of these stories from my biography as they are embarrassing, but they best demonstrate my behaviour when on clonazepam so should be included.

Walking home from the pub one night, I tripped and fell in the back yard where Dad parked the taxis. I had broken my arm with a spiral fracture of the humerus, leaving me completely immobile. Dad had been out on a hire, and fortunately, he saw me lying there as he turned to park the minibus up for the night. He and Mum helped me to the house where they left me to sleep on a downstairs couch. Still in a lot of pain the next day, the doctor was called out, and I was sent to hospital to have the break tended to. Unable to look after myself with my only working arm broken, I was once again shipped off to Adamson Hospital in Cupar to recover in one of their wards.

My stay was again for six weeks, and in that time, I "fell in love" with a charge nurse called Agnes. At ten years older, not quite five foot tall with blonde, bob-cut hair, perfect features and enchanting green eyes, she could easily have been ten years younger than me. She first came to my rescue when, while doing her rounds late one afternoon, I kept complimenting her on her amazing shiny teeth. Thinking this odd behaviour, she called a pharmacist friend and detailed the dosage of tramadol that had been prescribed by the hospital doctor. He told her to stop the drug immediately as the dosage was too high, meaning I was in overdose. She may have put me on a drip and made me drink water in an attempt to clear my system – a very vague recollection, because later that day, I had a seizure, confirming that tramadol should not be given to people with epilepsy, certainly not in overdose, and so I was switched to another painkiller.

Anyway, our friendship blossomed to the extent that, on one occasion, as she washed me in the shower, I dared suggest she get her kit off. Too much of a professional, sadly she did not, but she later told me that was the sexiest thing I'd said to her, so not entirely in vain. Before leaving the ward, I wrote her something of a love letter. The only bit I remember was calling her my Tammy, and when she came to ask what I meant by Tammy, explaining it was my teddy bear as a child. So I moved in with her and enjoyed a few months of the best *coffee*.

I'm not going to say all that much about our relationship as I remember Agnes with great fondness and only wish we'd met under different circumstances. I spent my days alone trying to set up a business as a website designer, renting an office in Lochgelly, with a grant from Business Gateway, and travelling there each day by bus. Agnes had just completed her degree and was about to start her master's, but I didn't want her to. Looking back, I can understand my selfishness, for she was an intelligent woman, and I was heavily sedated on clonazepam. There would be times I'd be sitting staring at the telly, not even watching it, and she'd have to shout to get my attention after my apparently ignoring her. For that reason, above all, our relationship was doomed to fail. Though not sure exactly why, I remember saying, "I have to go," and her sitting on the couch saying, "Okay," before giving me a lift back to Auchtermuchty. Having sent her a letter trying to patch things up, I received her reply a few days later and walked into the town with my jacket open, so the cold rain and wind would blow onto my chest as a means to punish myself.

I moved into my office in Lochgelly, with a computer and desk and chair for furniture, and a makeshift internet connection. I spent most of my time in the local pubs, one Celtic, the other Rangers, playing pool and drinking Guinness. By no means the west end, both pubs had iron bars on their windows as did all the local shops.

Eventually, the grant money for the initial rent of the premises ran out, so I had to leave. Not wanting to live with my parents again as I'm not the sort of person who can live in a restricted environment, I went to Fife Council, declared myself homeless, and they gave me a room in what was then the Tarvit Mill Hostel for the homeless.

It was spring 2005, I'd been watching the Champions League final in a Cupar pub, when I left in despair at half-time, with Liverpool 3–0 down, to walk back to the hostel. On arriving, they told me Liverpool had pulled it back to 3–3 and had gone on to win on penalties. To my relief, they let me stay up and watch the full game again as it was repeated in the early hours of the morning. Though I enjoyed living at the hostel and met some really nice people there, I was thrilled when eventually offered a flat at Langlands Road in St Andrews. I moved with great enthusiasm, believing life was taking a turn for the better. It wasn't the poshest part of town by any means, but even a rough area in St Andrews was paradise compared to where I'd been in recent times. *I'm not sure that it's drug related, but I never watch football now.*

Langlands Road was a council scatter flat (temporary housing), furnished with white goods, a bed and a settee. The single bed provided was too small so Mum and Dad brought over a double bed from their spare room.

I quickly established Aikman's Cellar Bar as my new local. Run by Barbra and Malcolm, along with a staff of students and local youngsters, Aikman's was the obvious choice, as they had live music at least three nights a week, and in my clonazepam years, I absolutely loved music.

I first met John and Jamie at Aikman's. A fairly chilled-out couple of guys, John explained that he was on weekend release from the nearby Stratheden mental hospital and hoped to soon be allowed to stay out of the hospital permanently. He said he was schizophrenic, having stabbed his mother to death as a young man. This seemed quite unbelievable, given his apparent calm and well-mannered nature – it would seem a testament to how medication *can* so profoundly help a person with mental illness. On getting to know John, he told me his chronic back pain was down to his parents punishing him by beating him across the back with golf clubs as a child. I have seen John in times when his doctors have tried to reduce the medication at his request, and he becomes very uptight, paranoid and a little aggressive, but given what he says is true, I could not condone such abusive treatment. John has been a good friend and often my only confidante when my own mental state was hanging in the balance, so I can empathise with his chaotic existence.

By far my biggest concern, when in St Andrews, was the letters from the Student Loans Company, constantly demanding that I send confirmation from the DHSS that I was still on benefits. It came to a point where I would recognise the letters when they arrived and hide them away in a bottom drawer, wishing they would stop. Then one day they called and offered to write off the loan – given my disabilities – and like a fool I said I wanted to pay the money back on getting a job. Of course, that just meant they kept sending out letters demanding proof of income, and when eventually, some years later, I called and asked if they would still be prepared to write off the loan, given my disabilities, they said they didn't do that anymore.

By explaining this, I'm looking to highlight my constant state of anxiety and inability to handle problems that would seem trivial to most.

Because I was living in a scatter flat, I was assigned a social worker to help me get settled in. On seeing how badly my leg tremors affected my dexterity, particularly when it came to housekeeping, she made a fresh application on my behalf for high-rate Mobility Allowance. This application was successful, more than doubling the mobility component, meaning an extra £100 each month for beer.

Which takes us back to Aikman's. It was here I met another amazing and quite unique character – Zoran, a refugee from the Balkans war. He was a brilliant storyteller, contriving tales of his escapades in South America where he got his PhD after having been expelled from UCL for unacceptable conduct. Unfortunately, I can't remember more detail, but they were wonderful stories, keeping youngsters entranced year on year. More importantly, he would often contrive to develop new cocktails for me to test free of charge. In these times, I didn't just drink beer or have a favourite nip, I drank pretty much everything in the bar, seldom having the same drink more than once in a night.

Aikman's had everything: great music, top-notch banter and some really hot barmaids. The first I took a shine to was Pea – very sexy, looking a bit like Jennifer Aniston and always full of energy. She had a boyfriend called Graham who I did not like at all, most likely because he was her boyfriend. Mind you, he and his flatmate did cut me a "line of coke" at one of their parties, later having a great guffaw at my expense on revealing it was chalk. I knew I should have just laughed it off, but I hated being made to look the fool – *the unseen shit that walks hand-in-hand with sedation.*

I don't remember much about our parties at Langlands Road other than they would start shortly after the pub closed and usually just involved sitting around getting more stoned. After some eighteen months, I met a guy called Charlie who was about to start a PhD in virology. Given the council were keen to free up the scatter flat, Charlie and me decided to share a place at 119 South Street. It was a large flat with very high ceilings, in a beautiful old building at the centre of town. There were to be so many parties here that someone actually scratched *Tony's Place* on the wall next to our door buzzer.

Not long after moving to South Street, I met a student in the pub who was doing a PhD in psychology, I can't remember his name, but he was ex-RAF. He told me about a project on facial recognition that was being led by his supervisor. Given my image-processing history, I contacted Professor Perrett, and he kindly gave me a chance, not an official position, just access to the lab to see what I could do. Working there made me feel I was a valued contributor to society, even attending in the weeks after breaking my big toe on the bath tap. Mind you, I also made it to the pub in the snow with a plastic shopping bag strapped to my stookie.

I had some limited success in the work but was having more and more trouble with spasticity in my left arm and leg when walking. My doctor suggested increasing the clonazepam from 1mg to 1.5mg a day, and much as this did ease the spasms for a while, it all but obliterated my already limited powers of concentration, leaving any further participation at the lab out of the question.

One day, when Mum was driving me back to St Andrews from Auchtermuchty, I remember saying it was just as well I wasn't allowed to drive, as I couldn't possibly maintain concentration. My sleep pattern changed as well, shifting from a reasonable eight to nine hours each night to one where I'd go to bed at the back of midnight after returning from the pub and sleep until three or four in the afternoon. I was effectively able to live in my dreams, manipulating what was happening as if it were real, only better.

We had countless parties at 119, so I should apologise to our neighbours for the incessant racket. Though the revellers were mainly students, others from the pub would attend. On Barbra's birthday, we gathered in the flat after closing time. Barbra, or Mum as she was better known, brought bottles of Martini and gin from Aikman's and, as I remember, sent someone back for more before the end of the night. I managed to get a band, Huge Mouse, my, and I think Barbra's, favourite at Aikman's, to come to the flat, where they would only accept travel expenses as payment. I believe some, including a particularly attractive university secretary, had their tops off and were dancing around in their bras, though that may have been another night. An offshore oil worker who drank with us occasionally at the pub had somehow got into the party uninvited, and because some of the girls found him frightening, as he was always high on coke, Charlie and John (or Stabber as Charlie often called him) took things in hand and removed him from the premises. Other than that, it was a fab night with the band playing long into the small hours.

Fiona (another hot barmaid) tended the cellar bar at Aikman's. With long, chestnut-brown hair, finely sculpted features and deep brown, melancholy eyes, a true classical beauty. Much to her relief, I am sure, she would never hear of my infatuation, though I did hear a friend of hers say, "Do you want me to speak to him?" and her reply, "No, just leave it," as I came in one night. Figuring she was perhaps unsettled by my constant attendance at her bar, and maybe wanted me to know she wasn't interested, I tried to vary my visits with the upstairs bar thereafter.

While Gordon, one of the cooks at Aikman's, was living with a very hot, young, blonde girl, another of our friends, Cameron, a psychology student, commented that their relationship would never last. According to him, she had daddy issues – it was textbook. Gordon was outraged on hearing this, and though they did eventually split, I certainly wouldn't want to venture a guess as to why. Cameron also told Zoran I would never make anything of my life as I was a drunken waster, also textbook. *I've not made much of my life as yet, but I gave up drink years ago, so you know where to put that textbook, laddie. Much as I found his comments annoying, they might actually have helped, instilling a determination in me to prove him wrong. So no hard feelings.*

I only had a brief encounter with actual carnal activity while in St Andrews and, sadly, I cannot remember her name, but I think I first met her and her brother at Tarvit Mill. Petite with blonde hair and happy, sparkling eyes, she attended one of our parties and slept with me that night before heading home the next day. She must have been quite daring, for it's doubtful that I'd have made an advance, though I was considerably more chilled on the higher dose clonazepam. It was just a one-night stand, but she did pop by some weeks later to say cheerio before moving to Glasgow.

Joe made a third appearance not long after the clonazepam dose was raised. A gay man came into Aikman's and groped me, saying, "Come out, for fuck's sake man!" Being so heavily sedated, I just stood there in shock. This may seem fairly trivial abuse when compared with the others, but if the same were to happen today, the perpetrator would find himself with a broken nose at the very least. *I should clarify that I don't necessarily have an issue with homosexuals, but I detest sexual predators, if that makes me a bigot then so be it.*

There are way too many crackpot stories from my time in St Andrews to tell them all here, so here's a brief summing up.

There were frequent trips to the Raisin to play pool with Ross, Martin and Charlie, where we usually ended the night with a kebab from the takeaway across from the student union. These kebabs were so good that one led to me being barred for life after farting in a pub on North Street.

There was the swine who ripped me off when I gave him £500 upfront to pay for a fab new laptop like Gordon's. And instead, he arrived with a ZX Spectrum-like contraption, which I did not accept, but I never got my money back. Then there were the times both Charlie and me had to break into the building as we'd forgotten our keys. I was lucky and got away with it, but Charlie had to pay for a new lock.

On the bright side, Johanna would often come round with her guitar and sing through the night. Occasionally taking us to the castle sands, where we'd build a driftwood fire on the beach, and she'd sing until sunrise.

I should also mention wee Charlie, another of Aikman's cooks. He was Irish, his actual name being Fergal, someone always full of cheer and cider. When deciding to leave St Andrews, I told him it was because I was doing nothing of value there, and he said I was wrong, that there were many who depended on me as the centre of our little community. This was a particularly kind and much appreciated sentiment, but it was time for me to go. Wee Charlie returned to Ireland not long after – all the best, old friend.

Shortly before leaving St Andrews, another Aikman's barman, a PhD student called Jamie Frew, asked what medication I was on. He explained there would often be times I'd come into the bar and sit staring into space in a complete daze, even before having a drink. He said I should type my medication into Google together with the letters "wiki" to learn more about the drug and its side effects. So, the following day I did just that. I won't go into the detail here, but the key points I learnt were: clonazepam should not be prescribed for longer than seven weeks to any patient who is not having multiple attacks daily, and even then, the drug should only be continued if it is highly effective at reducing seizures… a daily dose of 1–1.5mg will cause severe sedation. I could not believe what I was reading. Why had my doctors been prescribing me this drug for the past eight years?

It is not my intention to pass judgement on individual doctors, so any apparent condemnation here should only be taken as a reflection of my mindset at that time.

***

A couple of years down the road, I decided I wanted some compensation for having my career ended by clonazepam, so I wrote up my grievances and passed them to a law firm in Glasgow. I cannot remember the name, and because they went into administration a few years ago, I can't seem to trace them. Anyway, they agreed to take my case and arranged for me to meet with a consultant neurologist. He explained that, because I was initially prescribed clonazepam by a GP in England, and though he appreciated that had been inappropriate given she was not a neurologist, that charge would have to be brought to an English court.

As for me being left on the drug for so long, he suggested that because I moved around so much my doctors could not have known that my personality and behaviour had changed as a consequence of taking clonazepam. I argued that such a drug should not be given for more than seven weeks to patients not having multiple seizures daily, and he pointed out that, though he would agree, this was only an opinion and not sufficient to secure a judgement in law.

In conclusion, it was clear any attempt to secure compensation would most likely prove fruitless, so I left it at that.

***

We were refused a renewal on the lease at 119 South Street – it would seem that you can only have so many parties before the landlord tires of the complaints. Charlie decided to look for another flat in St Andrews. I really hope he succeeded in the end, for it would have been nigh on impossible for him to have completed his PhD had he continued living the party life at 119. Much as it may have slowed Charlie's academic progress, I hope he too holds some fond memories of our time there.

A friend of John and Jamie's called Ross Thom, who attended a few of our parties, tried to persuade me to share a flat with him in Cupar, but he'd always seemed way too "friendly" for my liking – the sort that shouts at you from across the street then comes running over to see how things are going when you barely know them. As it turned out, shying away and saying I needed a place of my own was a good call, because last year he murdered his ex-girlfriend, cutting her throat, before killing himself.

Unable to get a letter of recommendation from our landlord, and again homeless, it was back to Homes4Good, the council's new homeless accommodation squad in Cupar. Though posher, it was nothing like as homely as Tarvit Mill had been – not a place you'd want to be stuck long-term. Soon after moving in, I had a seizure in my room. When I woke, I was lying on the floor and unable to move as there was excruciating pain down my spine whenever I tried to lift myself. As it turned out, it was just a trapped nerve, but nonetheless, it rendered me completely immobile and unable to reach the emergency pull cord. I tried shouting, but the nearby rooms must have been empty, for I did not hear a soul for almost two days. When I finally did, I shouted as loud as I could, and a few minutes later, a warden came in and quickly called for an ambulance. I was put on a stretcher and taken to the Adamson Hospital to be X-rayed. They confirmed that nothing was broken before giving me dihydrocodeine to kill the pain. When I got back to the hostel there was a haggis supper waiting for me – I've never enjoyed haggis so much. I took dihydrocodeine for about a week and ibuprofen for a few more, and the pain eventually eased.

I hadn't been in the hostel long before finding a cottage at the Barony in Cupar. Though quite expensive – given I was now getting the high-rate mobility component of Disability Living Allowance, I could afford it. And so, once again, all my friends were yoked in to help me move. After moving to Cupar, John would come to my place once a month to clean. He would come down from the Stratheden Hospital after his weekly stint working in their gardens, give it the once over then take a bus back to St Andrews using his free bus pass. I would pay him £10, which he always insisted he didn't want because it made him feel good knowing that he was making a meaningful contribution to society, whereas his feeling good made me feel I was doing something worthwhile too.

On learning about clonazepam's side effects, I had confronted my doctor and insisted I was taken off the drug. Some months later, now settled at the Barony, I finally got an appointment with a neurologist at Ninewells. After being quite obnoxious in exclaiming my anger at having been prescribed and left on a sedative like clonazepam for so many years, she suggested Keppra, a relatively new treatment for epilepsy that had been seen to work in patients for whom all other drugs had failed. Then Dr Roberts, the consultant who had spotted the signs of a vascular malformation some twenty years earlier, came in and suggested that lamotrigine would be a more suitable drug given my tendency for anxiety. I asked if lamotrigine would sedate me, and when he replied yes, I insisted I would not consider another drug that caused sedation. He said that ninety per cent of his patients felt no side effects from their medication, to which I responded, "Nonsense! All drugs have side effects."

My apologies to both for my caustic nature that day. As I saw it, these drugs had ended my career before it even began. All the same, I would be interested to learn how Dr Roberts knew ninety per cent of his patients felt no side effects, given I was never, and still have not been, questioned on the side effects I suffered with any of these drugs. Anyway, it was agreed I be started on Keppra, two 500mg tablets each day.

Before moving to the Keppra era, it's worth noting that I soon got to know the pubs in Cupar. The Parsonage, run by Ian and Carol, became my new local, though, to be honest, I didn't particularly like either of them. The barmaids were Janice and Lynne; where Janice was the sensible, easy-going type you could tell your problems to, and Lynne was a scatterbrain who spent half her shift on the puggy. I chose the Parsonage because it was frequented by Malky and Jim, two extraordinary guys who would both talk of "the voices" and how they messed with their heads, though they never discussed what was said.

Malky was literally covered in piercings, with dozens of rings and studs in his hands, face and neck. He would often have fresh razor cuts on his wrists – the doings of the voices. Though Malky clearly had issues, I'd be best cheered on seeing him sitting at the bar when I arrived, because he was very easy-going and great company. Jim, on the other hand, or Jumping Jim as Janice called him, was likely cut from the same block as Zoran, though not as flamboyant. Where Malky cut himself to stifle the voices, Jim would drink. We all played for the darts team, none of us much good, though Malky was undoubtedly the best.

One darts night, there was no sign of Malky – only to be explained a few days later when Jim came to tell us he'd been hit by a bus when walking the winding country road back to his cottage in the dark. Some months later, he arrived back in the pub with all his piercings gone but looking pretty nifty all the same. He explained that his cheekbones and jaw had been smashed by the bus, so they'd had to cut the skin at his throat, peal it back over his face and replace the shattered bones with titanium implants before reattaching the skin. I have to say the scar across his throat where the skin had been pulled back suited him down to the ground – far more impressive than the piercings had been. .

I'm not sure if it was before or after Malky's shenanigans, but around this time, I met a revitalised minx – an HRT rookie – at The Parsonage. Our romance began as a one-night stand and only lasted a few weeks, with us actually going to the pictures in Dundee on one occasion. She had recently broken up with her husband, and though it was fun at first, she soon started telling stories of how she would lie crying on the floor at her work, even shouting and screaming because she was so upset – most likely explaining why she split with her husband. When she suggested moving in with me, I quickly ended things. Perhaps not surprisingly, Rachel was the only one who came back for break-up sex.

KEPPRA

As an out-and-out stimulant, Keppra was the exact opposite of clonazepam. From day one, it was like being on speed 24/7. No more the trauma of getting up in the morning, I was awake twenty-three hours a day and never felt tired. I spent my nights on the internet playing games and did three or four crosswords every day, including the *Telegraph*, *Courier*, *Express* and the *Record* – crosswords became my equivalent of having a job. On the minus side, twice a day, twenty-two and a half hours after taking each tablet there was an excruciating withdrawal. Always making sure I was in the flat at these times, I would lie on my bed with tremors in my chest as the tension grew in my shoulders, followed by about thirty minutes of agonising panic attacks.

I didn't report this to my doctor, thinking it just withdrawal from clonazepam, but as the months passed there was no let-up. No longer trusting my doctor's judgement, I reduced the dose to one tablet a day of my own accord, throwing away a second tablet each morning so usage would remain as expected. While this did not completely resolve the problem, it meant only having to bear one panic attack a day and getting a few hours more sleep each night. I loved feeling alive and full of positive vibes, sure there were great times ahead.

Some months later, having had no seizures, it seemed the epilepsy was finally under control, so I decided once again to give up drinking, longing for a car. There were two incentives for going back on the wagon: first, to save money, but more importantly, alcohol might interfere with the drugs and induce a seizure. Every few months, I would wake in the night in a frenzy, unaware of where I was, my heart pounding, muscles trembling and head buzzing, but this never progressed into a full seizure. On reporting these events, my doctors were at a loss for an answer, so it was recorded as partial-onset seizures – that being my best guess – and no treatment was offered.

Before switching to Keppra, I'd found a charity in Edinburgh looking for volunteers. Though a forty-five-mile commute, I had a disabled person's railcard, so I was working as a tutor, helping a group of unemployed, local youngsters learn to use computers. Soon, there was another Rachel, an autistic girl, who came to dominate my time in class. She was completely devoted to learning, constantly asking questions, eventually demanding all of my attention and becoming grumpy if I talked to the other students. She would get top scores in all the tests and seemed to benefit a great deal from the time we spent together.

The one negative memory I have of this time was walking from Waverley Station to the Old Royal High School at the east end of Princes Street where the classes were held. When starting, still on clonazepam, there were obvious erratic spasms in my left leg, and though it wasn't painful, I hated seeing people watch me walk this way. I had hoped the change to Keppra would fix this, but instead, the spasms got slightly worse.

In Edinburgh only two days a week, I needed something to do with the rest of my time so decided to teach myself to play one-handed golf. I fashioned a makeshift set of clubs, with irons, a driver and putter from Gordon Smith senior – a caddy at the Old Course – and new five and three woods from Auchterlonies golf shop in St Andrews. On joining the Cupar Golf Club, only half a mile from my house, I spent the rest of the week there and soon got to know a few of the older players who also played weekdays, occasionally playing with them but more often than not alone.

I was still playing dominos with the crew at the Parsonage, but drinking Coke or Irn Bru rather than alcohol – let's just say Carol (the publican) was not at all impressed. There were times when youngsters would mock my jerky walking – now worse with me sober – when we stepped outside for a smoke, but by December of 2009, having had no seizures in more than a year, I applied for a Motability car and, in mid-February, took my first driving lesson with a guy in Edinburgh. He didn't actually have a car that was set up for one-handed driving but did have an automatic and said he'd give me lessons anyway. First time out, he had me driving in the busiest part of Edinburgh, across the top end of Princes Street. Though I enjoyed the thrill, it was very difficult using indicators, the stalk being on the left side of the steering wheel and me only able to use my right hand, so after a couple of lessons, I decided to wait until my car arrived from BMW.

It was a 1 Series, automatic, space-grey, coupe, two litre TDI, M-type sport, with leather seats and a great stereo. First seeing her on 3 March 2010, I was over the moon. An engineer added a lever that switched the indicator and lights so they could be operated from the right side of the steering wheel, and Dad sat at my side as I drove back to Auchtermuchty and, eventually, Cupar. I had lessons from both Mum and Dad, my cousin's wife Sarah, David, Aunt Roggie, and one from Uncle Ken during which I drove through a red light in Kirkcaldy.

After working my ass off for the theory part of the test, having learnt all the questions and practised endlessly with hazard perception software, I scored one hundred per cent in the theory and ninety per cent on hazard perception at the test centre in Dundee. On 4 April 2010, with my parents on holiday in the Highlands, Ken took me to the DVSA centre in Kirkcaldy. Early in the test, a car came the wrong way down a one-way street toward us, and I slowed to a stop, letting him pass. Perhaps instilling some much-needed calm, for I relaxed, and the rest of the test seemed to fly by. Ken looked gobsmacked when I told him I'd passed with only three minor faults – I was finally mobile.

When I phoned Mum and Dad to let them know, I'm pretty sure they were expecting bad news, but they sounded delighted. That same day, driving to Edinburgh, fearless and excited to learn, I tested the car's speed on the road down from Kirkcaldy and going back up the M90, both times topping out at a little over 130 mph. I was speeding all the time – with my brain in overdrive, driving slowly felt unnatural and frankly, wrong – so I was constantly in minor accidents.

Within a few days, my foot slipped off the brake, sending me crashing through one of the bollards in a Tesco car park. Then a few weeks later, when flying down the road from Craigrothie to Cupar, on approaching the first sharp bend at the top of a very steep downhill stretch, while racing a Golf, I came into the corner far too fast, lost the back end and crashed into the verge, badly mangling the front and rear side panels. So the car was off to the shop again, and I was stuck with another courtesy car. Those being the only two shop-jobs for the first car.

My time was now spent teaching Rachel two days a week in Edinburgh, playing golf – having joined the Elmwood golf club after moving to a new and cheaper flat at 57 Crossgate – and exploring the Highlands, keen to see the best of Scotland. The cheaper flat was necessary because my disability money was now being used to pay the lease on the car.

At around this time, I was referred to Dr Sloan at the Cameron Hospital to try Botox (Botulinum toxin) injections in my left arm. The aim being to suppress spasticity, which not only made golf very difficult, but also induced counter spasms in my left leg, further impeding my already laboured walking. In the first instance, the Botox was highly successful, so I continued with the injections – occasionally making adjustments depending on the outcome of the previous dosage – every ten weeks for the next few years. Golf was a lot more fun without the constant jerks throwing me off balance, but for the last few weeks of the ten, the tremors would return. Ideally, I needed injections every seven weeks, but that was more than the NHS could manage.

Everything seemed to be going swimmingly when, driving back from Edinburgh one afternoon, on the road to Leslie from the M90 motorway, I decided I had time to pass the two cars in front and floored it. The back of my car slid across the road into the verge where it was thrown back onto the road, flipped onto its roof and slid to a halt. No one was hurt, and no other cars were involved, so it was just reported as an accident, being my fault. The car was written off, after only six months, with over 20,000 miles on the clock. A friend from the garage it was towed to later told me the back tyres were completely bald. So I had to wait for a replacement car to be built – another £30,000 worth.

I was caught speeding twice in the weeks before crashing; once stopped by a panda car, on the way home from Edinburgh, and a second time in a speed trap. Fortunately, I was just 14 mph over the limit each time, so only received six penalty points. I drove down to the central police station in Glenrothes and tried to persuade them I'd been overtaking a van the second time and so had to speed up. After going to check the tape, the sergeant said he could see no van. Then explained that some weeks earlier he'd been driving up to Perth when a car flew past him doing over a ton. He couldn't stop that car because he was off duty but knew he'd catch him later. I felt sick as a dog, knowing he was talking about me, meaning I'd have to resit my test for receiving six penalty points in my first year of driving. For some reason, I thought the DVLA might not notice, but of course, a letter came to confirm within days.

On 1 October 2010, one year after stopping drinking, I stopped smoking as a punishment to myself for getting caught speeding and crashing the car. As it turns out, the best punishment ever.

Giving up addictive substances like alcohol and cigarettes was perhaps made easier by Keppra. Though cigarettes were pretty tough, Keppra induced an absolute determination to succeed – one of the few positives that came with hyper-stimulating my entire brain. Alcohol was surprisingly easy, given I was nigh on an alcoholic, most likely because Keppra kept me on such an extreme high all the time, there was no craving for more. The hardest thing about not drinking was what to do instead. For years, whenever I took the train to Edinburgh, I would go straight to the bar at Waverley Station for a Guinness and play five songs on the jukebox. Then I'd cross Princes Street to Rose Street, and with one drink in each pub, see how far I could get before being refused service, or running out of cash, whichever came first.

After giving up drinking, I'd go to the Waverley Bar for a fresh orange and lemonade, play my songs, then head up to the Costa that overlooks Princes Street Gardens, for a large mocha. Much as this was nice, it was a long way to travel to sit alone with a soft drink (you can't socialise in coffee shops), so the outings to the capital had lost their charm. Even now, my biggest regret at having gone teetotal isn't missing the high but missing the company that came with the high. For though I revelled in the company of other drinkers while on the bottle myself, I find them sadly boring when sober, as I'm sure they would me were the tables turned. I miss socialising but can't for the life of me find a way around it. Alcohol may be the devil's brew, but it's not all bad.

When the new car eventually arrived, I couldn't drive it for a while, making me very tense and edgy. I got the bus to Dundee to retake the theory and hazard perception tests – passing with one hundred per cent and eighty-eight per cent, respectively second time round. David accompanied me to the road test – as the licensed driver – and on the way, we got into a massive argument because he wanted me to slow down. When we got there, he left and headed for home (sorry, bro). Now in a manic state of anxiety, I failed the test, and Mum and Dad had to come pick me up as I wasn't licensed to drive home myself. Getting a cancellation slot two weeks later, I passed with one minor fault.

Earlier in the year, before getting the car, I had decided to try for Microsoft certification by taking an online training course where there were experts available to answer any questions via text messaging. There were five disciplines, of which I got through the first four fairly easily, earning the qualification of Microsoft Certified Solutions Developer (MCSD), but I really struggled with the final exam – something to do with servers – needed for the Microsoft Certified Solutions Expert (MCSE) qualification. I took the exam a number of times and may have eventually passed, but I don't think so, for though it would seem unlike me to give up, I found system architectures really difficult to memorise. I'm pretty sure I settled for an MCSD and blocked out the fact that I'd failed the MCSE.

Anyway, in the months preceding the crash, I'd been building some software for the Edinburgh charity's office workers, using what I'd learnt when doing the MCSD – knowing no one would hire me unless I could show an example of my work, this seemed the ideal opportunity. It was just a windows app with a calendar, appointments and accounts management. On the days I wasn't working with Rachel, I'd go down to my den in the charity's main office at the Edinburgh University student union and develop the software using Microsoft C# – a truly awful compiler, but after some considerable hacking of its functions, I did eventually get a prototype, of sorts, up and running. Just as the software became ready for testing, I had the accident and was absent for several weeks.

On returning to Edinburgh after passing my test, I found the buildings all locked up at the Old Royal High School so went down to the student union, only to find the offices there locked too. One of the cleaners told me that the charity had folded, bankrupt, a victim of the Great Recession. She gave me access to the office so I could recover my computer, but that seemed to be that.

A few days later, I decided to drive back down to Edinburgh, hoping to find out more. Feeling really drowsy as I drove out of Leslie, the next thing I knew, a policeman was helping me out of the car, a fireman having cut the door open. He told me the car had lost traction on black ice, veered off the road and ploughed straight through a telegraph pole cutting it into three pieces. He said it was quite normal for me not to remember, given the trauma. As I was lifted into an ambulance, I spotted the computer, with my software on it *(the only copy)*, lying in the field – ironically, never to be seen again.

I soon realised he'd been wrong about the cause of the accident as my tongue was slightly bitten – but I kept this quiet, knowing I'd lose my licence if discovered. On increasing the Keppra dose back to two tablets a day, to prevent further attacks, I became hyper-stimulated – *I would say borderline psychotic.*

Motability's insurance company refused to insure me again on a lease car, but Motability would extend a loan. That, together with the £5,000 insurance claim for extras I'd paid for on the BMW, would be my only chance of getting another car. Mum came to the rescue, finding a black one-and-a-half-year-old Golf, two litre TDI sport, again with leather seats. Now a considerable liability, my car insurance was over £3,000 for the first year. To be frank, things did not calm, quite the opposite, as one might expect given my yet more animated state of mind.

Back to one hour of sleep a night and two panic attacks a day – it was a price worth paying for the freedom that came with a car. The Golf was very fast, and now that I'd lost the work in Edinburgh, I was spending more and more time on the road. Unable to restrain the need for speed, I would floor it as soon as I joined a motorway, always trying to prove my car was the fastest.

***

When living in St Andrews, I did sudokus every day, eventually graduating to *The Times* sudoku. If nothing more, it helped exercise my mind and gave me a sense of accomplishment. But after stopping clonazepam I became bored with sudoku and switched to cryptic crosswords, as I'd never understood how they were done, and I needed a challenge. There was a particularly sharp Bletchley Park old boy at the Parsonage who introduced me to "thinking outside the box". I'm not sure if he's still alive and sadly cannot remember his name, but I'd like to thank him all the same, for crosswords were to prove hugely important in keeping my mind at ease in the years to come.

Roger was another of the old-school regulars at the Parsonage, a grumpy old git from Ladybank, a bit like Frazer in *Dad's Army*. Though he was sure we were all doomed – when I gave him a lift back to Ladybank on a night of heavy snow and refused to take any money, he arrived at the pub the next day with a huge butcher's steak pie for me to take home for my tea. Sadly, as time passed, his emphysema worsened, and as he sat on the bench seat with his pint, he would struggle to catch every breath. Toward the end, there would often be faeces marks on his trousers, and whereas Janice would take a cloth and clean him up, Carol just barred him for life. A few weeks after being shunned by his only "friends", he was found dead in his flat, discovered by the smell of rotting flesh.

Every so often, in the years to come, when I was having real problems with my own sanity, Janice, Malky, Jim and me would meet at the Cupar Arms Hotel to play darts and dominos. I think because it helps to be with likeminded people in such difficult times, and Janice enjoyed taking care of the likes of us.

After years of suffering with arthritis, Janice came in one day and said she was going to try a radical treatment where they would destroy her immune system to relieve the pain. Though it did make a big difference, within a year, there was a cancer the size of a grapefruit in her lungs. She was convinced it was because she had no immune system now, and I reckon she was right, for the immune system is how our bodies naturally deal with cancerous cells, usually destroying them before they pose any threat (as best I understand it). When starting with my book, I tried to contact Janice, having not seen her in about five years, in the hope she might have some memories to share – only to learn that she passed away last year. I will do all that I can to protect my own immune system, in her memory. For only a fool does not learn from what others experience.

***

The summer after getting the Golf, I took a trip to Southsea to see Aunt Daphne, at one point racing down the M6 at 100 mph in torrential rain – utter madness. I still don't know how I survived. The seven-hour trip was great fun as driving was my main reason for going. Though a little hazy on the holiday itself, I do remember some snooker and fishing with Monty, and a day trip to Dover when, on joining a motorway, I raced straight to the outside lane cutting a guy off. He drew alongside in the centre lane and gave me the wanker sign, to which I returned the finger. This may seem a crude and unnecessary point to mention, but it perfectly illustrates my mentality at the time.

Initially, I intended to stop along Southsea on the way home after taking a girl I'd met online to Wimbledon – having been offered reserved debenture tickets for Centre Court by way of one of Zoran's contacts. Sadly, the tickets fell through, so I'd gone to Southsea first, but on leaving after a fab holiday, I drove up to London, having persuaded the girl to settle for lunch instead. As it turned out, she was severely anorexic and barely recognisable from her online profile picture, so after eating, I headed for home.

I've since had two further internet dates. The first with a woman about my age down in Sheffield. She seemed great fun online and very sexy, but on arriving, her having spent the morning on a sunbed, I was confronted with a woman so badly wrinkled through exposure to ultraviolet radiation she looked like a centenarian. We did have a good laugh at dinner, but later that night, when she came to my room in her lingerie, I could not be aroused. Which brings me to my final online date, where I met a girl in her late twenties at a Costa cafe in St Andrews. She didn't recognise me at first, but eventually came over to my table and asked if my name was Tony. We had coffee, and she suggested I update my online profile picture to something more recent.

My abiding memory of the Southsea holiday came on the road back, driving up the M6 in the outside lane. A BMW came racing up on my tail, so I pulled into the centre lane, selected sport gears and floored it. As we passed 100 mph, he was pulling alongside and at 115 mph was about to nudge in front when suddenly he fell away. Realising the Golf had slipped into sixth gear, I pulled into the inside lane and slowed down, happy to know this car was faster than the two I'd wasted.

***

Keen to retain my link with Edinburgh; on seeing an advert on Facebook for volunteer patients to be examined in medical consultancy finals at the Western General Hospital, I applied and was recruited, attending a number of times. With diagnoses ranging from Parkinson's to Cerebral Palsy, it seemed my low regard for the competence of our medical consultants – at that time – was well founded. However, in retrospect, it might just as soon be a measure of how profoundly Keppra was affecting my manner.

One of my biggest torments – that worsened with time after the brain surgery – was the spasms in my left arm and leg. Most common when nervous, they would burst into life whenever I met pretty girls in my Heriot Watt days, and similarly later with clonazepam – though then the spasms were more animated, particularly when walking. When driving on Keppra they were much worse. On getting excited and accelerating hard – when racing another car – my left arm would shoot into the air, shaking violently in spasm, thereby inducing an equally violent counter-spasm in my left leg. Though my doctor had increased the clonazepam dose to ease spasms while in St Andrews, I always believed the drugs were causing the problem in the first place. With the spasticity further intensified on the higher dose of Keppra, it was now clearly an effect of neural stimulants – but having no choice but to take the drugs, I had to find another answer.

Dr Sloan, the doctor giving me Botox injections, referred me to Ms McKechin at the Queen Margaret Hospital in Dunfermline, and she agreed to fuse my left wrist so the hand would no longer twist inward in constant spasm. At the same time, she would lengthen and switch the tendons in the hand, so the fingers would remain relaxed. I'm not sure about the wrist, but I remember having the tendon surgery while awake, using a nerve-pinching technique rather than anaesthetic – though she did have to revert to local anaesthetic for the thumb tendon. The wrist took a few months to heal, being particularly painful in the early weeks as I would not take opiates, but it was certainly worth having done, making a huge difference in alleviating pain and significantly reducing the frequency of spasms in my arm.

Then came the lone-wolf terrorist attacks by Anders Behring Breivik "against the Norwegian government, the civilian population, and the Workers' Youth League", where seventy-seven people were killed. Though having no interest in his politics, I understood how these lives held no value to him, that he was simply using them as a means to force people to listen. I could empathise because I felt much the same way about humanity, thinking humans stupid, worthless creatures. I didn't see myself as a mere human, rather I was a supernatural entity. Of course, I didn't voice my opinions, knowing they would not be well received – I may have been a psychopath, but I wasn't an idiot.

KEPPRA & LAMOTRIGINE

As autumn approached, I was finding it hard dealing with the panic attacks so asked my doctor for advice. He said Dr Roberts had also suggested lamotrigine, should there be problems with Keppra – a dose of 200mg per day, in the form of two 100mg tablets, to be taken together with the 1,000mg of Keppra. In retrospect, it's obvious this was an error. The 200mg dose of lamotrigine was suggested as an alternative to, not in addition to, Keppra. Taken together, the doses should have been 500mg Keppra plus 100mg lamotrigine. Which in itself would have been too much as I can only tolerate seventy-five per cent of the minimum recommended dose with any anticonvulsant. This botched prescription was twice the dose recommended by the neurologist and 2.67 times the maximum I could tolerate, and so the mania went manic.

Shortly after taking the first of these tablets, I was driving to Anstruther and almost passed out on the road. Still very woozy on reaching the town centre, I scraped the passenger door along a lamp post when turning down a side street. Though really struggling to concentrate, I made it back home without further incident and was able to get Millrat to patch the car up a few days later.

The drowsiness quickly eased on getting used to lamotrigine. Instead, I now got an erection immediately after taking a tablet and was horny all day long. The effect intensified whenever I took a tablet thereafter. For the next few months, I spent almost all my time on the computer looking at porn and masturbating, losing interest in almost everything else.

After chatting to a woman on an online dating site, she sent me a photograph of herself lying naked on a bed with her legs spread wide. When working in the City, she'd had back trouble and was prescribed clonazepam, the same dose I was initially on for epilepsy. But the financial work had become too much, and she now ran a burger van. When I messaged her the side effects I'd learnt about before coming off clonazepam, I could almost see her turn white with shock. And not long after, she disappeared from the dating site. Here's hoping she got her life sorted out. If she is, by chance, reading this, she need not worry, for though very attractive, I deleted her photo about a year ago. Sure it was clonazepam lowering her inhibitions that motivated her to send the picture, I didn't feel right keeping it.

A few weeks before changing my prescription, I'd contacted Manuel, now a professor at Dundee University, to see if there was any chance he could find me a research project. Now that he had, and I'd agreed to join his lab, something had to be done about my obsession with porn. I asked my doctor to change the prescription from two 100mg tablets to eight 25mg tablets – allowing me to spread the dose across the day, so I wouldn't have such a high on taking each pill. Though this helped a little, I had to further reduce the dose to six 25mg tablets before the porn obsession abated. However, with six tablets, I would start to have panic attacks ten minutes before the next tablet was due, so I increased the dose to one tablet every three hours and forty-five minutes. But though this did stop the panic attacks, I was now very unstable.

The memories I hold for my time at Dundee are patchy, only recently coming back to mind after being suppressed by a beta blocker called propranolol for five to six years. On top of that, I was always in a hyper state of mind while at Dundee and so would seem to have fairly good recall of significant events but little for the mundane. Moreover, it is difficult to attribute names to the people I was working with. Mind you that was also true when I was at Dundee as I forgot the name of my professor at Ninewells, a Professor Houston, a few months after first meeting him. I will report things in turn as I remember them, doing my best to form an accurate timeline.

The project Manuel found for me was very exciting. The idea being to build a piece of software that would construct a 3-D model for a full-body MRI of blood vessels, then automatically search for and identify varying degrees of stenosis (narrowing of the vessels), with the object being to enhance detection of such lesions and reduce the processing time for these enormous images. On doing some background reading, we agreed on two possible solutions for the first stage of development, settling for Manuel's preferred choice. Adria, a Spanish postdoc who had already got things underway with the project, had written a paradox on a whiteboard, and even after he explained that it could not be solved, I spent days trying to unravel it. The one crossword I really struggled to make sense of back then was *The Times* cryptic, so on getting one two-thirds done, I left it lying on my desk for months, believing the others would think me clever for managing so much – a measure of my faltering lucidity and confidence.

For Christmas, our department would put on a show for school children in Dundee with the aim of encouraging them to take up science. It was a very flamboyant affair, with Manuel as the star, and though he tried to persuade me to take part, literally trembling at the very idea – now a nervous wreck – I outright refused.

I was soon introduced to Jane, a PhD student about to start her first year. I imagine she was feeling a little overwhelmed by what she was taking on when she told me it was a refreshing change to find someone in this very serious business taking a 'light-hearted' approach. Before long, I was invited to share an office with her at Ninewells in Prof Houston's group. I loved working there, for the project was progressing well, with pretty impressive results from the outset, at least in the sense that they looked great, and though I wasn't actually being paid, it did feel like a real job.

I'm not sure about the timing for this next story, but it must have been early on, because I was only invited to attend one conference while at Ninewells. It was a lecture by a prominent brain surgeon (I think) at Glasgow University. I drove three other students down to Glasgow, and after a hectic battle with TomTom telling me to go up one-way streets in the city centre, I eventually gave up trying to find another way, and did as TomTom suggested.

Initially, Jane sat with me in the lecture, and though having little if any real understanding of what was being discussed, I decided to ask a question, trying to link what he'd been talking about to my brain surgery. On hearing his answer, I asked yet more questions. I was behaving like a child and am really sorry to have caused Jane such embarrassment, but that's how drugs like Keppra and lamotrigine work on me, somehow lowering my inhibitions. For the second half of the lecture, Jane wisely sat elsewhere, and though continuing to raise my hand with questions, I was not given a second chance. We had something of a hectic ride back to Dundee, and though driving "slowly" to suit them, we did have a hairy moment on approaching one of the roundabouts on the outskirts of Perth. That was the last conference I was invited to – I assumed at the time, because of my driving, but though feasible, I'm sure that was not the primary reason.

Jane had taken a year out of medical school to give her mother palliative care two years previously and was having some difficulty with depression now, so she decided to ask her doctor about treatment. She was referred to a psychiatrist in Dundee, and for several weeks, I would drive her up to see him and wait for her in the car until they were done. It was only a few visits and things were quickly sorted out, but she seemed worried others would find out, for back then, there was a stigma that surrounded depression.

After about six months, we attracted funding from an MRI software company based in Edinburgh, sadly I can remember neither its name nor the name of the person we dealt with. The lab was upgraded to include two new state-of-the-art PCs with loads of memory for handling the huge data files – meaning I had all the computing power I could ask for. I would set test runs going at the end of the day, and often travel back up to Dundee in the middle of the night to check results, sometimes coding into the night. I was absolutely obsessed with the work, and being unable to sleep, this seemed to be the best use of my time.

In the day, I would go down to an old railway carriage on the south side of the Perth road, not far from Dundee Airport. Here, I would buy two bacon and egg rolls and a can of Irn Bru, then park up by the river, where there would often be seals lying on a little island at the foot of the Tay rail bridge – though at the time, I preferred to concentrate my attention on crosswords, as they seemed to help keep my mind in check. As time passed, I became less comfortable with being in Dundee so would cross the river, stopping at the little snack bar on the far side of the water to get a bacon and egg roll and hotdog with onions before continuing to a lay-by en route to Tayport. I knew of this spot because I took that road each day when travelling to and from work so as to avoid the temptation of speeding on the dual carriageway.

This is where I first noticed the panic attacks and tachycardia after eating. My first instinct was it had to be down to the anticonvulsants, given they would seem to have been the source of all my past troubles. But as the weeks passed, I realised that excess salts, acids, sugars and spices, in my diet, noticeably aggravated the symptoms. Indeed, cutting dietary stimulants to an absolute minimum would have been a makeshift solution – though not one suited to someone in my animated state for I could not resist the high that came with eating such foods.

Apparently of the mind that a fresh conundrum would help alleviate these troubles, I became infatuated with Pea back at Aikman's Cellar Bar in St Andrews. I would often pop in to do crosswords when I knew she would be on shift, for she was exceptionally good, solving *The Times* cryptic every day with consummate ease. She did get me a ticket to come see her in a show at the Byre Theatre – where with me seated to the right of the centre of the house, as her and the other dancers turned and pointed to the audience shouting "you", they all seemed to be pointing at me. Though probably just my imagination, given she invited me, it seemed plausible.

Whatever the truth, my anxiety left me incapable of managing relationships of any kind, and given what was to come, it's as well it ended there. In the weeks and months that followed, I continued to pester her from afar on Facebook and Messenger until eventually being blocked. There's no way to undo history once it's written, no matter what the reasons, and that truth will always haunt me.

Our Christmas party that year was a very posh affair at one of the choice hotels in Dundee. When I picked up Jane, as her escort for the night, she was wearing contact lenses. This being the first time I'd seen her without glasses, she looked quite stunning as she stood waiting at her door in an evening dress. We had a lovely meal and some laughs with the crowd from the Department of Medicine at Ninewells. I had a couple of small ports from the bar, trying to calm my nerves, but the effect was minimal. This was the first time I'd felt a strong attraction to Jane, but unlike my obsession with Pea, my foremost desire was to make her happy, not for her to make me happy – it was a magical feeling.

The next day, I gave Jane and her boyfriend (I cannot recall his name) a lift to Edinburgh Airport, from where they would fly to Ireland for the Christmas holidays. Now thinking of her all the time, my obsessive behaviour switched from Pea to

Jane; it was an awful Christmas. I would race the car around north-east Fife every night, once passing a car at 110 mph going around a blind corner. My reasoning being – if there had been any vehicles coming the other way, I'd have seen their lights. Of course, had there been a cyclist on the road, they would have been killed, but I didn't think of that. Again, the reason for this madness was that I could only relax when driving fast and taking risks, and with the ever-increasing stress over Jane, it was getting worse by the day.

About this time, my trips around what I called the Anstruther loop (exit St Andrews taking the Grange Road past Kinaly to Anstruther and back by way of the coast road through Crail) increased to almost daily. I would wait until well past sundown, so I wouldn't have to worry about police and would be able to see cars coming by their lights. The road was perfect for racing with several chicane-like sets of Z-bends and a number of good straights allowing for speeds of up to 100 mph.

Though there was a thrill in driving so fast, I was not thrill-seeking; rather, I was using the thrill to suppress the unbearable anxiety that was crippling my mind. I took Barbra's daughter, Sarah, and her fiancé, Chris, on this trip a couple of times. I like to think their second thrill may have somehow contributed to Sarah becoming pregnant, as the two left my car full of vigour.

Before writing my story, I had some considerable concerns about confessing to illegal driving and what the consequences might be. However, given that in the four years driving while on Keppra, I had an accident every few months, and in the eight years since, I haven't been involved in a single accident, I don't see how anyone can reasonably argue that I should be held responsible, and even if they do, it is more important that the effects of these drugs become public knowledge.

After the Christmas break, I picked up Jane and her boyfriend from Edinburgh Airport. They seemed full of cheer, having had a great holiday, and though jealous, I was just happy to see her again. They invited me to their flat for drinks the following Friday to thank me for the airport runs. With thick snow on the Dundee roads, I drove her boyfriend to the shops to get supplies – racing down one hill so as to have enough speed to get up the next, a hair-raising experience, but we somehow survived.

I'd brought weed with me and ended up sleeping on their spare bed that night – because I was stoned or because of the snow, I'm not sure which. But I left early the next day – for as the cannabis high waned, seeing them together and hearing about their capers in Ireland had lost its charm. I must have gone to see them at the flat more than once, because I remember driving back another time very stoned – something I certainly wouldn't recommend as it was quite terrifying.

Having just broken up with his girlfriend and looking for a fresh start, Martin, an old drinking buddy from the St Andrews days, came to do a nursing degree at Dundee. One afternoon, when giving him a lift back to Cupar from St Andrews, I asked him if I was going too fast. He told me to stop the car. I did. He snorted a line of coke and said, "I'm fine. Carry on, lad." *The coke brought him temporarily onto the high I was on all the time – and so he could handle the speed.*

One morning, Martin was late and he asked me for a lift so he wouldn't miss his first class. Though tending to stick to back roads to avoid speed traps and the impulse to race other drivers, on this occasion I made an exception, taking him the fourteen miles from my flat to the university in less than ten minutes.

Though my trips with passengers never led to an accident, there were plenty all the same. There was one where the car spun 360°, after running over the kerb to avoid a Land Rover coming around a corner on my side of the road. Fortunately, the Golf survived, only needing minor bodywork repairs.

I bumped into the back of a car when a young girl stalled at traffic lights in Dundee. I told her I didn't have my insurance documents with me and instead gave her my phone number, saying I'd pay for the damage if she let me know the cost. She texted later that day saying that her father was angry I hadn't given her my insurance details and the repair was around £160. I immediately transferred the money, and she thanked me for being so honest.

Another time, when racing back from St Andrews, I overtook one car – only just scraping past on the narrow road – then stopped just short of a Tesco van with my brakes hard on. The van had to reverse as there was a car coming the other way across a narrow bridge – but because I was so close behind, there was no time to get out of his way, and he dinged my front bumper. The driver came out to get my insurance details, and as we were talking, the guy I'd overtaken stopped on passing and told him I'd been driving dangerously earlier. There was only slight damage to my bumper, and I told him I'd rather fix it myself, as I didn't want to claim on my insurance. He said that should be fine as there was no damage to his vehicle. He just needed my details in case I filed a claim against them.

Not long after – when on the dual carriageway heading for the Tay Bridge – I decided to weave my way through the traffic, overtaking on the inside then bouncing off the side of a white van on my way back to the outside lane. I turned off at the next roundabout and fled toward Tayport. The van followed initially but soon gave up the chase. I drove straight to the police station in Cupar to report the incident, saying I'd come off the road at the roundabout so we could exchange details, but he had not followed. I told them I didn't know where the police station was, when they asked why I'd not reported this in Dundee. I don't know what made me think this would help, other than it's a crime to not report an accident. Fortunately, nothing more came of it.

Of course, the cost of repairs for all of these incidents came out of my pocket as, with my insurance premium still around £2,800, I could not afford to make claims.

Each of these past two days when recording what happened on Keppra, my whole upper body was trembling as if the muscles were somehow remembering how they felt every day back then.

Back to August of 2012. When reversing into a parking bay in St Andrews, so I could pop by Aikman's to see Pea, a taxi driver told me I couldn't park there because that space would become part of a taxi rank at five o'clock. I told him I would only be five minutes, and to get out of my way, because he was standing in the middle of the road by my car door. He then said I was parked on his foot. But I was sure that wasn't possible, as he was standing by the door and the wheel was further forward – then a taxi driver friend of his shouted, "You're on his foot!" as he appeared from behind the car. They both seemed pretty aggressive, so I ignored them, reversed back into the space and nipped into the pub. I left for Dundee five minutes later and thought no more of it.

Some seven weeks later, the police arrived at my flat to arrest me. However, they did let me drive my car to the Glenrothes police station where I was handcuffed, fingerprinted and had a DNA swab taken – with the understanding that these would be destroyed if I were not charged. The charge was assaulting a taxi driver in St Andrews. They explained that I'd been accused of parking my car on his foot. Reading from Mr Dukes' (the taxi driver's) statement, they related pretty much the same story I've told you, only adding that once he told me my tyre was on his foot, I deliberately turned the wheel before reversing back. I admitted to everything other than parking on his foot and turning the wheel – insisting I was simply trying to park, and given the taxi driver had no jurisdiction there, continued to do so. They accepted my story, and no charges were brought.

A few weeks later, I received a letter from a solicitor in Dundee to inform me that a civil case was being brought against me for causing injury to a Mr Dukes. The claim was for around £4,000 against my insurance company, and they wanted to settle. But I refused to settle and tried to engage a lawyer myself. He agreed to take the case – on the understanding we could secure legal aid funding – but my application for legal aid was refused on the basis that my insurance company had agreed to represent me for free. The fact that they were not prepared to defend me was irrelevant. So I decided to represent myself and attempted to build a defence – highlighting what I saw as inconsistencies in the witness statement and taking photos to show that Mr Dukes foot could not have been under the wheel, given where he was standing.

A few days before the court hearing, my insurance company's lawyer called to let me know Mr Dukes currently had another case outstanding where he'd accused another driver of parking on his foot. I told Pea at Aikman's this, and she said Dukes was a rogue and a chancer, always involved in one scam or another, leaving me confident I would win.

We were late getting started on the first day, so had to return to the court a few weeks later for the final arguments to be heard by a different judge. On speaking to my insurers' lawyer during a break in that session, he seemed confident I'd completely discredited Mr Dukes and his witness. Nevertheless, we lost, and the insurance company had to pay out, which meant my insurance rose to £4,200 for the coming year.

Of course, my account of this time is based on memories, and given that I was not of sound mind, by my own assertion, it's possible I've somehow subconsciously distorted the facts in order to remember what I would want to have happened rather than what actually happened. I had come to hate Mr Dukes with a ferocity I'd never felt before. Again, I am certain this was down to the medications, for I feel no hostility toward him now.

At around Easter 2013, I asked Prof Houston to arrange for me to see a neurologist, in the hope we could find a more suitable anticonvulsant. On meeting a consultant at the Perth Royal Infirmary, I did my best to explain the situation – without being too explicit, afraid I might lose my licence – but in retrospect, that was never going to be enough detail. He said the only alternate treatment available was lithium. Luckily, I knew John had been taking lithium for many years, as an antipsychotic. It destroyed his memory, leaving him barely able to concentrate at times, and I was not prepared to sacrifice my mind in that way.

One night, after leaving Ninewells in a very agitated state, I continued past home and headed south, driving at breakneck speeds to somewhere on the east coast about twenty miles south of Edinburgh. I can't be sure how far or exactly where, but while driving at around 90 mph on an A road in the dark, there was a flash in the rear-view mirror. Quickly coming to my senses, figuring it was a speed camera, I turned the car, slowed right down and headed back north. A police car joined the road at the next roundabout and followed me for about five miles before breaking off and heading back south. I told Jane about this, and she seemed quite shocked, asking why, but that's just a hazy partial recollection.

My final car crash came about when driving to Kirkcaldy on the dual carriageway from Glenrothes on a very bad winter's day. I was following a bus in a lane that had been ploughed when I decided to overtake. On moving into the fast lane, the car started bouncing on chunks of ice, eventually spinning around and crashing into the central barrier. I wasn't hurt, but the car was in a bad way, and after assessment by a garage, the cost for repair was going to be more than half the value of the car, so my insurance company wanted to write it off. This time, my brother came to the rescue, saying that him and my nephew Connor would do the job for whatever the insurance company was prepared to pay, and given he is a qualified panel beater, they were happy to go with this. The two of them did a fantastic job, far better than I could ever have expected. I doubt that I'll be able to repay this favour so a big thanks to them both.

While the car was being fixed, the work continued to go well, but my attraction to Jane was becoming a real problem, so much so, I was asked to meet with her supervisor to discuss the matter. I don't remember exactly what I'd been doing or saying to upset Jane – not having access to those memories – but I do remember insisting the problem was with my drugs, and that as things were, I could not continue without her.

KEPPRA

Later that day, I made an appointment with my doctor to see about changing the medication. Given it was overcharging me sexually, the obvious solution, as I saw it, was to try stopping lamotrigine and increase Keppra to three tablets a day, one every eight hours, in the hope the increased frequency would mean daily minimum levels would be high enough to stop the panic attacks. She said, "You always seem to manage your own epilepsy medications anyway, so yes, why not give it a try."

I cannot find words to adequately communicate how misguided that advice was.

So I did, and it worked, in that the panic attacks stopped that same day, but thereafter, I was on cloud nine. It was absolutely amazing; every woman I saw looked stunningly beautiful, even those I'd had no interest in the day before. Later that week – while Jane was at a conference in America – Prof Houston came to my office to do an appraisal of my work. Delighted with the progress, he seemed confident we could get funding for me, rather than just the travel expenses I'd been receiving, and that we could have a research associate and PhD student join the project. I was absolutely thrilled and quite literally as high as a kite, so my recollections of that day may be somewhat distorted, but I cling to them for this is the closest I ever came to achieving real success in my work.

The following day, sitting on the bus en route to Ninewells, feeling hot air from the heater blowing up my trouser leg, I was sure it was God entering my body, and believed that I was the chosen one. So I texted Jane in America, telling her I loved her, and that everything was going to be fantastic, or words to that effect. Only to come crashing back down to Earth on reading her reply: *Have you lost the fucking plot?*

LAMOTRIGINE

The exact timing of what came next is hazy. I do remember being moved to the room outside Prof Houston's office but not much after that. I tried to come to terms with what was going on, but soon gave up, as my mind had become so chaotic I could no longer function. The only option left was to try switching to lamotrigine.

Cold turkey withdrawal from Keppra was by far the worst I've experienced on stopping an addictive substance, leaving all else to pale into insignificance by comparison. With all my muscles trembling, and crippled by overwhelming fear, I would have signed myself into Stratheden Hospital for mental healthcare, had I not been sure they would suspend my driving licence. Instead, I took to smoking cigars in a desperate attempt to calm my nerves.

Once, in the early morning, when leaving the flat, I looked back at my stuff as if for the last time. Then I drove to a nearby road where I could reach well in excess of 100 mph and smash through the stonework at its end. On reaching 115 mph, the car went into sixth gear, and I relaxed, so I turned back for home. *I don't know why speed made me feel so good, but I'm thankful for it now.*

The following is a letter from my doctor asking the mental health nursing officer at Dundee University to see me in mid-July. It suggests that the change to lamotrigine had fixed the problem, but given I didn't feel any guilt and the perversions persisted, though less emphatically than when on both drugs, it would seem this was a ruse concocted by me in an attempt to convince the university I was well.

Ms Grant

I would appreciate it if you would see this 45 year-old. He suffers from epilepsy and was treated for more than 5 years with Keppra. He describes some quite dramatic side effects from the Keppra as the drug was increased. He describes having "fantasies of seeing women naked and cutting off their genitals and eating them raw". Also fantasies of cutting off their heads. Since he changed his drug to lamotrigine he has not had these fantasies but feels guilty about them. He doesn't have any auditory or visual hallucinations and no thoughts of harming himself or anyone else. He seemed quite agitated and keen for some help to come to terms with this. I would be grateful if he could be reviewed and assessed.

I note that Keppra can have quite significant CNS side effects and that it is good that he has stopped it, however I feel that he will benefit with some help to assist him with the feelings of guilt and maybe some tools to help him deal with it.

After my meeting with Fiona Grant, the mental health nursing officer, she reported her findings to Dr Watson as follows:

Dear Dr Watson

Thank you for the updated information confirming your agreement to reactivate this man's referral, further to his department manager contacting me I saw him on 23.07.13 for assessment.

In fact, Mr Doull attended out of courtesy only, having refused the previous offer of contact in early March 2013. He did not believe that he was unwell nor in need of associated input.

He denied any previous psychiatric history, stating that he had never been referred to mental health services in the past. He related all his problems to various medications he'd been prescribed since 2000, but (as per your letter) most notably Keppra, which he states he was taking simultaneously with lamotrigine.

He described and cited disturbed thoughts re killing, hurting or mutilating others in terms of varying degrees of insight over time. He denies ever acting on these at any level and discussed these thoughts with significant deprecation at interview. He reported marked changes in his functioning over the previous four weeks since changing medication. Although there had been some residual agitation initially, that had subsided after two weeks and he was by this point, feeling very optimistic regarding his progress.

He stated that he did not wish to discuss his family history at interview, so I did not gather this information.

Mental State Examination

There was no evidence of impairment in concentration, motivation, interest or enjoyment levels. His mood was euthymic, no agitation nor specific anxiety featured and there was no thought or perception disturbance apparent.

I did not elicit any current evidence of risk to self or others in our contact.

He was focusing on his study related projects, regarding which he reported much sharper concentration, far greater creative thought and productivity, with optimism about his future prospects. He was aware of ongoing feelings for a female colleague about whom he had been preoccupied, but realised and accepted that these feelings were not reciprocated and so had made arrangements to remain working in an alternative location, to avoid further discomfort to both of them. He had made no attempt to contact her in recent weeks.

He described a fairly solitary lifestyle outwith work, living alone and having no intimate relationship. However he does visit a local pub regularly for social company, although continues to abstain from alcohol, having previously drunk to excess in the past. Mr Doull was quite content with his social situation at present, wishing to continue focusing on his career and stabilising his health.

Impression and Plan

Although still a little upset at his recent experiences particularly, Mr Doull did not present with any manifestations of ongoing illness, his previous difficulties apparently having alleviated further to medication changes. Both reported and observed functioning did not support the need for psychological input at this time.

We therefore agreed that we would make no further arrangements for contact, but that Mr Doull could contact me for review, should that be indicated in the future.

Having forgotten I'd asked my doctor to refer me to Fiona in July, rather thinking I'd gone to see her on the first referral in March, I got in touch recently to ask for a copy of my case file – keen to learn what I'd told her at the height of the crisis with Jane. However, I think these later interactions are still worth recording.

Over the coming weeks and months things got even worse. On several occasions, when driving, I got severe pins and needles in my right arm, and once, when walking up from the park in Cupar, my right leg collapsed, first on the steps coming out of the park and again at the top when I fell to the ground. A couple walking past offered to get an ambulance, but I got to my feet and insisted I was okay, while thinking it had be something to do with lamotrigine.

Fearing it may have been a prelude to a seizure, I increased the lamotrigine dose from six to ten 25mg tablets a day, and so there was a significant escalation of my perversions. I started downloading scat-eating porn, where naked women eat each other's stools, and I remember masturbating while watching a phone video of a Mexican man cutting off a woman's head with a knife. Also, there was a recurring fantasy where I would cut Mr Dukes' genitals off and force him to eat them. I know some people are naturally aroused by images such as these, but in me, it was definitely drug-induced, for I don't get turned on by obscenities like this now. *Sorry for having to be so explicit, but only with the entire truth can you hope to comprehend the poisonous effect these drugs had.*

When my mind seemed a little more balanced, I did try going to Manuel's lab, to where my computers had been moved, with the understanding that I continue working from there for the short term at least (I worked in the evenings when the others had gone home, for I could not yet face them). When doing a test run one evening, I remember saying out loud, "I need to know if you are there for me. If you are, the result for this test will be 568." – the result being the number of features found in an MRI image, where the average was between two and seven hundred, and the majority were between four and six hundred, so you might say, a 200–1 shot. When the result was 568, I remember feeling sick and trembling with shock, not knowing what to do. This was the only time I ever asked such a question, as I was before and am now an atheist, but on this night, I became convinced otherwise. After going home for supper, I drove back to Dundee and wiped all the computers of my data, keeping a single copy for myself.

This is where my ego went supersonic – I was sure I could force Ninewells to take me back, because I was irreplaceable, and, with a divine force behind me, unstoppable. It would seem I was using the supernatural as a coping mechanism to manage a situation that I simply could not deal with otherwise.

Not long after, having failed in my attempts to force my way back in, I built a website hosted on an American server and used it to present all the work I'd done at Ninewells. If memory serves right, I was expecting someone to offer me big bucks to bring it to them. I did put a link to it on my Facebook wall, but I'm not sure anyone ever visited the site, and after a year with no one having contacted me, I decided it wasn't worth paying for its hosting, and www.seeingstenosis.com was no more.

Toward the end of November, while making supper, there was a sharp pain in my chest. On calling NHS 24, I described my symptoms to the operator, and she asked if I could get to the hospital myself – at which point I exclaimed, "Fffuuuccckkk, it's getting worse!" She told me to try to relax and sent an ambulance. By the time it arrived, I was on the steps outside my flat, unable to stand. The paramedics were very calm and reassuring, saying they'd better take me to hospital just to be safe, as they carried me to the ambulance. On the way, they stopped once, on seeing a strange arrhythmia on their monitor, but it stabilised, so we carried on. The paramedic came in with me to explain what he'd seen to a nurse, and shortly after, I was taken into surgery. They gave me diazepam and, while looking at my chest with a scanner, fed a wire in through my arm. I was given a second diazepam when it got sore, and in what seemed like a flash, the job was done.

The surgeon had found what he described as a ninety-nine per cent occlusion in my right distal coronary artery, just after it leaves the heart, so he'd cleaned it out and put in a stent. I was taken to the ward and prescribed tablets (including: ramipril, statins and a beta blocker) – as I understood it, to be taken for the rest of my life. This was explained by a young intern, but still quite sedated, I don't remember much of what he said.

That night, I woke twice with the feeling a seizure was starting. It was like the partial-onset seizures that started with Keppra, only now my head was turning to the left, as it had as a child – but still, they did not progress to a full grand-mal seizure. I was released the following day, having had an ultrasound scan that portrayed my heart as grossly normal – meaning there was no apparent damage.

Mum and Dad took me to live at their house for the next few weeks. I was smoking those vape things, rather than cigars, to help me deal with the anxiety. As the days passed, the partial-onset seizures continued, so I further increased the lamotrigine dose to twelve tablets a day or 300mg (twice what I could tolerate). Of course, the sexual obsessions got even worse. I was hiding away in my bedroom all day long, downloading pictures of naked women. It was so bad I would masturbate, ejaculate and continue to masturbate without loss of erection. I shudder to think what might come of it, should Billy Connolly get wind of this.

Though a tad embarrassing, these exertions may have been key to my heart's recovery… it's an ill wind that blows no good.

Eventually, one afternoon I had a seizure while exerting at the laptop and, on waking, decided to find out more about the heart drugs prescribed by the hospital. On reading up, I discovered that sixteen per cent of people with epilepsy will have a seizure induced if they take ramipril. I wasn't prepared to give up my licence for a year because some idiot doctor prescribed a drug that caused me to have a seizure, so it was not reported. On stopping both ramipril and vaping, the partial-onset seizures immediately eased, and I left my parents' for home, finding it hard to care about anything.

Some months earlier, Manuel had got me an interview with the company sponsoring our work at Ninewells. I drove through to Edinburgh extremely spaced on the lamotrigine, got lost and eventually arrived about an hour late. The interviewer kindly saw me anyway, but like earlier interviews, back when I was on clonazepam, I had no idea what he was talking about and could barely answer any of his questions. Nonetheless, I was obliged to Manuel for trying so hard to help, even given my insanity, so I told him about the heart attack and made some effort to apologise for my behaviour, sending him the project data back should anyone want to use it.

I made hundreds, if not thousands, of posts on Facebook during my time at Dundee. Initially, in trying to court Jane – before she blocked me – and later, expressing my indignation at being "forced" out of Ninewells, with yet more covering withdrawal from Keppra. Throughout that time I was so erratic, I would make a post in the morning, then delete it later in the day, horrified I'd said what I had. Though I do remember changing dozens of these posts to "me only" viewing on my Facebook timeline, when I checked, hoping to use them to help document what happened, I found nothing. I made my first attempt at an autobiography about a year after leaving Ninewells – while on lamotrigine and propranolol, a beta blocker (I will explain later) – but I eventually gave up, unable to concentrate on writing or make any sense of my life. It would seem I then decided to delete these posts, in an attempt to cut my ties with the past and make a fresh start.

Throughout this hellish turmoil, there was one shining light, and it may well have been my monthly lunch dates with her that kept me on the rails. Johanna, the girl who used to come sing through the night at 119 South Street in St Andrews, had returned from Sweden in 2012 to do a master's at Edinburgh. I'm ashamed to say, I'm not exactly sure what subject she was taking, but it was probably related to the business of putting on festivals, concerts and the like. We would meet every month, more or less, in the best of Edinburgh's eateries. I'd always been attracted to Johanna, for she had the most beautiful eyes and made me feel comfortable in her company, being kind and supportive where no one else was interested. I was reassured by the fact that a highly intelligent and beautiful woman was prepared to dine with me and listen to my inane drivel.

We continued to lunch for about a year, trying out many fine restaurants. The top three for me being: The Museum, where the view looking down on the castle was absolutely stunning, and though learning that I don't like sea bass, the food was very good; the Castle Terrace Restaurant directly below the castle, not far from Princes Street Gardens, where we had lobster followed by a teensy pudding that looked very disappointing when it arrived, but the chocolate was so rich and delicious that on finishing I didn't need more; and number one would be The Kitchin where we had something like five courses – the one I remember best being an enormous mushroom, which Johanna recommended, having picked the same wild in Sweden. I feel my mouth watering now, as I remember its juices bursting over my taste buds. Then we had partridge and pear, and pudding was a chocolate orange with dark chocolate covering a bitter-sweet orange truffle. There were also little taster bites between courses, some sublime freshly baked bread, a tantalising cheese board and great coffee.

Much as I loved these trips to Edinburgh, the road home was always uncomfortable with my left eye twitching, the left side of my face going numb and an occasional panic attack. Looking back, this was an effect of too much anticonvulsant, where the symptoms were aggravated by eating sugars, spices and fatty acids (in the likes of whole-grains, vegetables, fungi, cheese, lobster and sea bass) – but I had no idea what was happening at the time.

When I started this section a few days ago, I found my upper body was trembling at the end of writing sessions, but now

I've made my account, this has eased. It's as if by telling the stories, however horrific, and rationalising my understanding of what actually happened, the trauma has abated.

***

By late spring 2014, I'd gained three stone in weight and was so weak that after showering in the morning I had to take a rest on my bed before drying myself. Always short of breath, I was never able to get enough oxygen. I also found my head was becoming unstable, not as bad as with ramipril but occasionally turning to the left when driving, as if I was about to go into seizure. Again, I did some research and found that the beta blocker (I don't remember the name) would likely be slowing my metabolism and causing the weight gain, while at the same time lowering my blood oxygen level by turning off beta cells in my lungs – so I weaned myself off, knowing my heart had been categorised as grossly normal after the heart attack.

As for the head-turning, this was a little more complex, but I learnt that around twenty-five per cent of the body's cholesterol is used by the brain to keep its cell membranes stable, and that "good cholesterol" cannot penetrate the blood/brain barrier. Given that statins stop the liver producing the "bad cholesterol" the brain needs, they were effectively starving my brain of vital "fuel". This might be fine for a person with a normal brain, but for someone like me, it sounded very dangerous, so I stopped the statins as well, and within days, the episodes had eased considerably, stopping completely within a month. *Remember, I'm just explaining what I did and why – my reasoning may well be flawed.*

My condition's complexity had apparently changed, for now there were two similar types of attack to contend with. The first being partial-onset seizures as was described with ramipril and, to a lesser extent, with statins, where my head turned to the left in the way it did before going into seizure as a child. Then there's what I thought was insulin shock – a blast of adrenaline where I would wake staring forward not knowing where I was with my heart racing and muscles trembling. If this was indeed insulin shock, it could have triggered a grand-mal seizure in the years before getting my epilepsy under control. These attacks, though similar to the twenty-two-and-a-half-hour withdrawal, as was described earlier with Keppra, always started while asleep or falling asleep.

I thought this might be down to an insulinoma (a benign tumour producing insulin constantly) which could be removed with surgery or, perhaps more likely, reactive hypoglycaemia where the pancreas makes too much insulin when having a high carb meal, and not enough glucagon (a hormone that causes liver cells to release stored glycogen when blood sugar falls too low). That, and because I'd seen House deliberately put himself into insulin shock, where the way he looked as he returned to consciousness was exactly how I felt as I came round after an attack. *When referring to "insulin shock" hereafter, I mean a partial-onset seizure – where I would wake staring forward, not knowing where I was, with my heart racing and muscles trembling – that I thought (hoped) was triggered by low blood sugar.*

Having lost some of the weight by summer and feeling stronger with my blood pressure back to normal, I decided it was time to get my life sorted out and make a fresh start. Never having settled into a proper job, I'd never had the chance to get my personal finances under control, so debt had been a burden throughout my adult life. When first leaving school, the Bank of Scotland gave me a £4,000 loan before I headed off to university in Glasgow, then a further £3,000 on switching to Dundee. Neither was ever repaid, as was also true of my student loan from the Heriot Watt days – around £15,000. On top of that, I owed Sky TV £500 and Scottish Power £2,700 from my time at the Barony and 57 Crossgate.

Before moving to pay-as-you-go meters, the only time that I paid utility bills was when working in Weymouth, so there will certainly be more due. Because my only income is from state benefits, that being the minimum allowance the government decrees I need to live, I could not be forced to repay these debts. There is a token amount of around £6 a week that can be deducted from benefit payments, but having learnt this years earlier, I made sure to not pay my council tax up front, so the council got their money a year in arrears, which meant no one else could get money from me through the courts. I figured my tax was eventually paid to the council, so felt no shame in this.

Not long after moving down to Weymouth, Mum and Dad had contacted me to say Granny Doull had been in touch to ask if I would mind her giving the money Grandad had left for me when he died – thinking I'd need extra help being disabled – to my younger cousin Johnathan, to be used as a deposit for a mortgage on a house in Norway. Much as I was reluctant, given it would have cleared my debts, this being the first time I'd heard about the legacy and knowing that Johnathan was much closer to my grandfather, attending his church sermons every Sunday for many years, it seemed only fair that he should get the money.

Now sickened by the constant letters from debt collectors and feeling repressed by my inability to secure any sort of credit, I approached Citizens Advice to ask for help with setting up a repayment plan for these debts. They explained that, because I live on benefits, paying off the debts would make no difference to my credit rating – just as it is accepted that I don't have enough money to repay old debts, it is assumed that I cannot afford new. Feeling completely helpless with no apparent hope of bettering myself, I gave up on the idea.

A few days later, on finding a bulging wallet in the men's toilet at the Parsonage bar, I took it through and gave it to the barmaid – I think it was Lynne – and when she asked the patrons to check their pockets, one of the old boys jumped to his feet. Having just picked up his pension that afternoon, he seemed very relieved and handed me a fiver, insisting I take it. Later that week, I was approached by Lynne's best friend, Maggie – who occasionally worked as a relief bartender at the Parsonage – and was invited to join the North East Fife Credit Union as a director. Initially, I volunteered as a teller for a collection point at the Girl Guides' hall in Auchtermuchty (an hour a week) and attended a directors' meeting once a month in Cupar. Now, though having made no effort to pay off my debts, I had access to credit. I remember thinking, *Is it any wonder there was a financial crisis?* I Continued to work these shifts for the next three years, and though relatively trivial, it did at least give me some sense of self-worth.

Now having completely lost faith in my doctors, believing them to be responsible for all that had gone wrong in recent times, I decided to contact Professor Perrett at St Andrews University – hoping he might offer to help, given I'd once worked in his perception lab. Wrongly believing him to be a psychiatrist, I sent a huge email describing my problems. I will not include it all here, but the following two paragraphs from that email help reveal the extent of my psychosis:

I started working with Prof Manuel Trucco and Prof Graeme Houston at Dundee University in December 2011, developing software to automatically detect stenosis in full-body MRI vascular skeletons. Initially things went well, my mind was fairly stable and the work was progressing well. However as time passed I started having feelings for a girl I was working with, I decided I had to increase the level of lamotrigine as the anxiety was becoming bad

again. I did this on consulting my doctor. The obsessing continued to grow. Now taking 300 mg of lamotrigine a day I started having terrible nightmares and sexual fantasies where I would eat women's genitals, cutting them from their naked body and frying the flesh in a pan beside the bed as they watched. Often I'd cut my penis off and fry it for them to eat.

After a time the girl made it clear she wasn't interested, I became very depressed, desperately trying to find a combination of the drugs that would solve my problems. I decided, on agreement with my doctor to stop taking lamotrigine and move to 1.5 grams of Keppra, taking each of the three pills four hours earlier each day to stop the 22.5 hour problem. Things seemed to be going well, the come down was no more and I was very happy. I started having fantasies where I was kissing the girl from work. One Saturday night I lay on my bed for 6 hours imagining we were kissing; sure she was doing the same. I was trembling with excitement throughout, adrenaline pumping through my body. Eventually I climaxed in what seemed like ecstasy, a feeling I cannot describe, though I did soon tire of it and went back to the kissing.

Professor Perret did not reply to my email, so I drove to St Andrews to ask if he'd received it. He said he had but was sorry for he could not help; I would have to consult with a doctor. I'm really sorry to have burdened him with this madness and can only hope he won't think badly of me for it.

A few months later, still lost for an answer, I sent the following email to my MSP with the certainty that, given the dangerous driving, he would arrange for me to see a psychiatrist.

Dear Mr Campbell

I hope you won't mind me contacting you directly but I think you are my only hope. I've tried to be brief in my description of the problem.

Back in 2000, shortly before I started work with the MOD as a research scientist, a GP from Southsea changed my anticonvulsant (taken to control epilepsy) to clonazepam. My progress thereafter was laboured; I left after 18 months for a PhD studentship at the University of New Hampshire, believing the lack of progress in my work was down to the inefficiency of DERA. After eight months I returned from the States having spent the majority of my time there partying at the local bars. On returning to Scotland I applied for many jobs, travelling across the UK to attend interviews. Of course I wasn't successful; Clonazepam causes severe sedation as would have been obvious when interviewed. After several failed attempts at setting up my own business, and times spent in homeless hostels I became aware of the side effects associated with clonazepam via Wikipedia. One being that doses from 1 mg to 1.5 mg as I was taking, cause severe sedation and prescription should not be continued after seven weeks unless in the severest of cases where the drug is highly effective. In 2008 I insisted my doctor take me off the drug immediately. He said the effect of clonazepam on my mental health had not been realised because I'd moved around so much, and the doctors hadn't the chance to get to know me and understand my condition before starting on the drug. The consultant neurologist at Ninewells confirmed they seldom use clonazepam to manage epilepsy now, and so they switched me to Keppra.

Keppra made me very uptight, a withdrawal 22.5 hours after taking a pill was very severe, I'd go to my bed for that hour, and lie trembling and in a state of panic. I came to realise this was down to the Keppra and not withdrawal from clonazepam, but I hadn't had a seizure in six months, so I decided I could live with this. Six months later I got my first car through Motability. I would often find myself driving across Scotland at 120+ mph because the anxiety was so severe, it seemed this was the only way I could relieve the tension. I wrote off two brand new BMW's in my first six months driving. Fortunately no one else was hurt when I was high on this drug. In the summer of 2011 my doctor prescribed an additional anticonvulsant lamotrigine to help alleviate the anxiety.

I started working with Prof Manuel Trucco and Prof Graeme Houston at Dundee University in December 2011, developing software to automatically detect stenosis in full-body MRI vascular skeletons. Initially things went well, my mind was fairly stable and the work was progressing. However as time passed I started having feelings for a girl I was working with, I decided I had to increase the level of lamotrigine as the anxiety was becoming worse. I did this on consulting my doctor.

In the end I realised I had to come off Keppra, I had a complete mental breakdown in withdrawal. I was asked to leave the project and my funding was withdrawn because of my apparent obsession with the girl. I won't go into detail, suffice to say no action was taken by her or the university, but once again I found myself unemployable because of anticonvulsants.

Earlier this year I published my work on the internet. To be honest I wasn't fully settled on my new drugs at the time, and so I'm not sure it's well presented. I'm leaving it there as is (a legacy of my time on Keppra). If you are interested you'll find the work at "www.seeingstenosis.com".

I just want people to know what these drugs can do. My consultant told me that another of his patients had to be sectioned under the

Mental Health Act Scotland when he was given Keppra. Yet in 14 years I only saw a neurologist once, in 2008 to change my prescription to Keppra, and I've never had any psychiatric care. With psychiatric care we'd have realised clonazepam was sedating me, and given that it never controlled my epilepsy there would have been no reason to continue the treatment. As for Keppra, again it would have been obvious the drug was causing harm, I should never have been allowed to drive when on Keppra. I was a danger to myself and others.

"People with epilepsy are three times more likely to commit suicide than the general population, and women with the disease have a greater suicide risk than men, according to research in Denmark. The Danish study is not the first to link epilepsy to an increase in suicide, but it is the first to use a comprehensive, nationwide population registry to investigate the association. Newly diagnosed epilepsy patients were more than five times more likely to commit suicide than patients who had been diagnosed more than six months previously. A 29-fold increase in suicide risk was seen in newly diagnosed patients with a history of psychiatric illness."

I want to draw your attention to the increased risk, 3*5 = 15 times that for the general population, for patients in the first six months after diagnosis. This is the period when they are first prescribed anticonvulsants. Given that I've flirted with suicide when overwhelmed by these drugs I cannot understand why no psychiatric care whatsoever is given to patients with epilepsy, particularly when being introduced to new drugs. Instead the government plan to reduce the basic care offered. People who are given antidepressants are far better cared for, and those drugs are less dangerous.

I would ask you to report what happened to me and try to convince the government that more not less care should be provided for people with epilepsy.

My apologies for the earlier version of this email, there were a couple of points I missed.

Best Regards

Anthony J. Doull

He replied as follows:

Dear Mr Doull

Thank you for your e-mail of 30 December with regard to your concerns about epilepsy medication and the unfortunate side effects that it has had on both your work and personal life. I would strongly encourage you to remain in regular contact with your GP and advise

them immediately of any side effects that you
believe are a result of your medication.

I have now written to Shona Robison MSP,
Cabinet Secretary for Health and Wellbeing,
and Dr Brian Montgomery, Interim Chief
Executive of NHS Fife, with regard to what
support is available for people with epilepsy,
and I have attached copies of this
correspondence for your information.

I would hope to receive responses from Ms
Robison and Dr Montgomery in the near future
and will be sure to forward them on to you as
soon as possible.

Yours sincerely,

Roderick Campbell MSP

I did receive a further response, from someone high up in the
NHS, saying that there were two neurologists available for me
to consult with in Fife, and little else. Not much help, given
I'd completely lost faith in neurologists.

Now off Keppra, my sleep pattern had completely changed.
But whereas the beta blocker had left me tired all the time;
now, about an hour after having dinner, I'd get really tired and
go off to bed – at around five in the afternoon – and sleep
until early morning. As I saw it, there were three possible
explanations. First, my heart – though apparently normal after
the stenosis had been removed, perhaps there was some
permanent damage. Second, there was my earlier self
diagnosis that my pancreas was making too much insulin –
where low blood sugar would be making me tired. And

finally, lamotrigine – though known to cause tiredness when changing dose, this was persistent and no worse after taking a pill, so it seemed unlikely. Lamotrigine was a lame duck explanation, because there were no alternative anticonvulsants – that I knew of – so it was ruled out.

In the coming year, I tried changing to a heart-friendly diet, but all those recommended made my face numb, induced heart palpitations when falling asleep, and panic attacks became a problem again – this time just a tight feeling in the back of my neck with my heart racing; it was quite frightening, especially when it happened at night. I did make another trip to hospital by ambulance, after severe heart palpitations in the night, but this "brush with death" was a false alarm.

A few months later, my annual blood tests identified chronic kidney disease – so, perhaps all my troubles were down to my kidneys not filtering my blood properly. Inspired by the chance that we might finally have an answer, I had an ultrasound scan done, but of course, the kidneys were found to be normal. *Blood tests now show that my kidneys are fine, so I never actually had 'chronic' kidney disease.*

Deciding to just eat food that caused no problems, I would have Lorne sausage and chips for tea, with no more than a can of Coke and one bar of chocolate a day – because anything more meant heart palpitations became a major issue. Convinced the problem lay in my head not my heart, I decided to join Falkland Golf Club, playing eighteen holes every weekday come wind, rain or shine – my new life goal being to become good enough at one-handed golf to play in competitions. But anxiety was a serious problem as it's really hard to play a smooth golf swing with tense shoulder muscles. On consulting with my doctor, she suggested propranolol, a beta blocker that's often prescribed to people with epilepsy in an attempt to alleviate anxiety caused by anticonvulsants.

After some experimentation, we settled on 80mg per day, and this really seemed to help, particularly at first.

However, in the months to come, the Botox injections were becoming less and less effective, until eventually, they made little or no difference. Beginning to suffer a lot of pain in my right shoulder, aggravated by the paralysed left arm wrenching against my swing while in spasm, I decided the only answer was to have the left arm amputated. So I made an appointment to meet with Ms McKechin again. When I asked her to cut off the arm she'd earlier fixed, with the main reason being it was impairing my golf swing, she seemed hesitant but arranged for me to put my case to the Edinburgh College of Surgeons. On explaining how badly the arm was impeding my play, one surgeon asked if I could not just play other people with a matching handicap. I told them there were no others, and it was not only that I didn't want to settle for a higher handicap – the left arm's spasticity was damaging my right shoulder. They were very considerate in listening to my arguments, eventually agreeing amputation might be a final option but asked me first to meet with Professor Hart in Glasgow, for he had developed a new technique for severing nerves which effectively did the same as Botox, but the effect would be permanent. I reluctantly agreed and soon had an appointment with Prof Hart.

On my first trip to Glasgow Royal Infirmary, I took the bus, thinking it would be difficult to find parking in the centre of Glasgow. A two-hour trip each way, there are two stand-out memories. First, just before arriving at the hospital, a guy got on the bus. He had the majority of his left arm amputated, his right hand amputated, and one leg partially amputated above the knee. Apparently mentally retarded, he was waving what was left of his arms around and laughing. Shocked, having never seen anyone like him before, there was considerable relief in knowing I wasn't about to have my arm amputated. The second memory is from the return trip. Our Glaswegian bus driver was full of cheer, saying he'd just been granted visas to move to Australia. He explained that they'd wanted to go for years, but hadn't been able to because of family ties here in Scotland. When a passenger asked what had changed, he replied, "The wife's mither died on Saturday."

At the appointment, Prof Hart explained that he would separate the nerves into strands, where half carry sensation signals, and the other half are for movement. They can tell which is which as a small electric charge will cause a movement strand to twitch the muscle. In the first instance, he left a small number of movement strands along with those for sensation in the hope this would allow some movement but not enough to trigger spasms. Though fine at first, the nerves quickly regenerated, and so these were later completely removed, keeping only sensation strands to retain a sense of touch. This worked well, but it took a number of operations over several years to get things just right, and as it turned out, by the last of these, I'd been forced to give up golf as my right shoulder was so badly damaged I could not risk further disabling my only working arm.

The only later development was in finding a way to stop my left arm banging into my leg when walking. Because there's almost no muscle left in the shoulder and bicep, my left arm lies flat against my body, meaning I needed something to push it back out to where it would naturally be. I took an old bar towel, folded it in half along its length then rolled it around an elasticated strap that loops across my chest and around my back to hold it in place – with another strap over my shoulder to pull it up under the armpit. I then stitched the towel, creating a towelling tube, and filled its centre with short pieces of plastic hosepipe, so forming a solid cylindrical mass, about six inches long with a three-inch diameter. When in place, the arm is pushed out from the shoulder, swinging freely as I walk, preventing the hand from hitting my thigh and triggering leg spasms – significantly improving both speed and posture.

***

I did try to enrol in a trial for a cholesterol drug at Ninewells, but given I'd already decided lowering cholesterol by reducing the amount of "bad cholesterol" produced by the liver was not suitable for me, it would seem my real motivation was that I was missing Ninewells and hoped I might somehow rekindle a connection. Going to radiology for the enrolment blood tests and form filling – only a few yards from where I'd once worked – was an eerie feeling. As it turned out, I had a minor infection, and so they said we'd have to postpone starting for a month. I asked the nurse if she would call me when they were ready to try again, and she said she couldn't, for they weren't allowed to badger patients, but if I contacted her in a month, she'd run the tests again. Not having enjoyed being back at Ninewells as much as I'd expected, I decided to leave it at that. As it turns out, a very good decision, because another drug in the mix would have yet further complicated my search for an answer.

There is another earlier vague "memory" where, in responding to a volunteer project at Ninewells, I let them take an MRI of my brain for use in research. Though I can see the radiology unit, which I knew from my days working in the adjacent Department of Medicine, I cannot picture the inside of the MRI machine. Then I remembered Jane had volunteered to have an MRI scan done of her brain, to be used in research, and realised this was just a dream from my days of longing to be back at Ninewells.

Having failed so profoundly while at Dundee, I became totally obsessed with demonstrating that I was not an idiot, and so decided to figure out *The Times* cryptic crossword, this being the one I had always found most difficult. Getting *The Times* every day for the crossword alone, I spent several months devoting all my time to it; being sure I fully understood every answer and checking the next day for anything not solved. Whenever lost in understanding an answer, I'd check with my friends on Facebook where usually someone could help. Once I got the hang of things, I posted my solution on Facebook each day, with the answers all explained, for two months. Though seeming a bit ridiculous now, it did help boost my confidence, and gave me something to do.

One day, back when on Keppra, the police had come to my door to ask if I'd been sitting in my car at the East Lomond car park the previous day. I told them I went there most days to do my crosswords and asked why they wanted to know. The female officer said, "It's nothing to worry about – some people have overactive imaginations." On another occasion, I was there at 1 a.m., again doing a crossword, when the police arrived. This time they said they were concerned that I might be suicidal but left, happy with my explanation that the epilepsy drugs kept me awake all night, so I came up the hill to do crosswords and enjoy the breathtaking view, rather than be stuck indoors at my flat.

Though now able to sleep better on lamotrigine only, I was becoming more and more isolated, forced to live a solitary life on the fringe of society. Then one afternoon, while at the East Lomond doing my crossword, a yellow Labrador pup came rushing up to the car to say hi before taking off up the hill. I decided then I needed a companion, and that companion should be a yellow Lab. I'd been searching for a while when Mum found one, only twenty miles away, at Loch Leven. It had just been listed on Gumtree, so I phoned immediately, and they said they'd keep the yellow female pup for me to see an hour later. The pup was only four weeks old, and I fell in love with her immediately.

She was registered as Bobby McGee, named after the girl in Kris Kristofferson's song 'Me and Bobby McGee'. I clearly remember worrying that she might not like me, so either my arrogance had abated or I actually cared. In the coming weeks, I prepared for her arrival by buying plates, food, a plastic bed with pillow, etc., thinking of little else. On 30 August 2015, Mum came with me to pick her up, holding Bobby on her lap as we drove back. Mum and Dad insisted on paying for McGee, saying they had some money they wanted to give me anyway and thought this would be the best way to spend it. When we arrived back at Cupar, Bobby tore into the flat, immediately laying claim to her new home. After a lot of racing around, she climbed onto the glass undercarriage of the coffee table and spread out as if deciding that would be where she would sit from now on.

Dad came to pick up Mum, so I wouldn't have to leave Bobby alone, and we spent our first night together. She would have none of the notion that she should sleep in the plastic bed, but rather stood, banging her two front feet on the floor until I lifted her up onto mine.

The people I bought her from had called to ask me to come pick up Bobby a couple of days early, as they'd not been able to get a vet's appointment, so her first inoculations would have to be done by my vet – but as it turned out, I couldn't take her before Sunday anyway. She did seem very excitable when we arrived to collect her, and Mum mentioned this to one of the girls – but she'd said, "It's no wonder given…" then paused and said something like, "…fighting with the other pups." On Monday, when taking Bobby to the vet for her inoculations, we found the real reason why. Her left eye tooth was snapped in half, with little more than the root remaining. John, our vet, got us an appointment with the only vet dentist in Scotland, down in Musselburgh. This time, Dad came with me to hold Bobby as she would need general anaesthetic. We left her with the dentist for an hour or so, and on returning to pick her up, she started barking immediately on hearing my voice when I talked to the receptionist, so all was fine. The cost was partly covered by a month's free Kennel Club Insurance that came with her, but I had to pay an excess of around £300 as the extraction was over £1,000.

In the coming weeks, Bobby could be an absolute trial, getting almost manic at times, so I watched some episodes of *The Dog Whisperer* in search of an answer. He explained that when they go manic, they think they're the boss and so can do as they like with no need to respect a master. The solution is to hold them on the floor, on their side, with one hand on their shoulder so they can't move. Eventually they calm down and go completely still, and when you lift your hand, they go to lie quietly in a corner by themself. The first time I did this, it was absolutely heartbreaking to see her go lie on her own, but eventually, she worked up the courage to come back over and lie quietly on my lap. You should only ever have to do this once to establish the pecking order. Though I had to do it three times with Miss McGee, it worked in the end.

Another issue was, though Bobby quickly learnt not to poop in the house, she did not learn not to pee. Indeed, sometimes she would walk across the living room not knowing she was peeing. During those first three months, she was up at least twice every night with me getting dressed and taking her down to the garden from the first-floor flat where I now lived at Westfield Avenue in Cupar. After several visits to the vets for UTI tests, courses of antibiotics and setting a special eating plan, we were still none the wiser, so she was referred to the Dick Vet Small Animal Hospital in Edinburgh.

Leaving her at the hospital for treatment was an incredible wrench; I'd never felt anything like it before. But of course, the opposite was true when I returned to pick her up two days later – as I sat waiting in a small consulting room, she arrived at the door and, on seeing me, peed all over the floor and jumped straight up onto my lap.

The vet explained that they'd done a number of tests on her bladder and found a very high concentration of white blood cells in the bladder wall. The only case that matched her symptoms exactly was a dog in Canada that had gotten a parasite in its bladder and developed allergies to all the food it was given thereafter. Apparently in such cases, the immune system assumes that dietary proteins it does not recognise are causing the problem and so it attacks them rather than the parasite. The dog in the one documented identical case was fed shortened protein biscuits for the rest of its life. But Bobby hated shortened protein biscuits, refusing to eat them, and given she would eat absolutely everything else, they must have been pretty vile.

I will return to Bobby's diet in the next chapter, but first, I must address what was happening with my anticonvulsants during this time.

There were two further critical side effects with Keppra and lamotrigine. The first became apparent almost immediately on starting Keppra: a belief that I was getting younger, perhaps in part because I was so full of energy, never tiring, filled with the same revitalised certainty of great things ahead I'd felt as an adolescent. But it was more than that, for people much younger than me now looked old. As I understand it, the teenage brain is pretty chaotic with all its functionality working in overdrive, and as we age, some of these fall away to be eclipsed by the dominant traits that define each individual's adult mind. With Keppra switching everything back on, my brain reverted to its adolescent state, so I *had* become younger but not in a good way. *(It was several years after the Keppra prescription was stopped before a natural balance was restored).*

The second, becoming more effeminate in my manner, was perhaps more down to lamotrigine. Emma, the girl I used to play pool with at the Hollies, mentioned this on Facebook. I assumed she thought I might be gay, but she said, "No, your *behaviour* is feminine, posting all your problems on Facebook, always wanting to talk things out, things men just don't do." And she was right, for I certainly wouldn't now. On top of that, I was nervous and highly strung, not a trait in all women by any means but certainly more prevalent in women than men. Now a nympho teenage girl in his mid-forties – what else could possibly go wrong?

Back to when I first got McGee. By the end of the summer, my porn obsession had reached the point where one day I found myself clicking a link to Catholic schoolgirls being belted. As I did, a *Police Scotland* message appeared on the screen. I panicked – partly because propranolol made me so paranoid – deleted all the porn that I'd downloaded, which was all legal anyway, formatted the parts of the disc where the images had been stored and cancelled my subscription to Three Mobile Broadband, later changing to BT, in the desperate hope no one would ever find out I'd tried to access that site. There was a button I could have clicked to say that I'd clicked the link unintentionally, which would have been much easier, but I was sure that was some kind of trick.

It was then I realised that I had become *Joe*. Beta blockers may reduce sex drive normally, but they made no difference with me when on lamotrigine. So, I went to my doctor and told her about my fantasies of cutting off women's genitals and eating them while having them do the same with mine – not daring to mention the Catholic schoolgirls for fear of being locked up. No longer prepared to live with these perversions, I insisted something had to be done, and was referred to the Victoria Hospital in Kirkcaldy.

In the weeks to come, the panic attacks when driving got much worse; probably because I was trying to minimise the dose of lamotrigine. For example, as we drove down to the harbour at the East Sands in St Andrews, it would start, always at the same place, with adrenaline pumping through my body, my shoulder muscles would go rigid so I couldn't move my head, and there was trembling down my spine. I was sure it was adrenaline as I'd had the same sensation, to a much lesser extent, ever since my dentist started adding adrenaline to my local anaesthetic.

Some ten weeks on, there was still no word of an appointment from Kirkcaldy, so I phoned the hospital, and the receptionist told me it wasn't listed as an emergency appointment. I told her that, if I didn't have an appointment within a week, I would stop taking the lamotrigine. And within a couple of days, I had an appointment for the following week.

I was very concerned about my ability to concentrate and that I wouldn't remember what I wanted to say when meeting the neurologist, so I prepared this letter to read to him:

I'm asking you to consider changing my epilepsy medication from lamotrigine to a drug with less side effects. These include: anxiety, palpitations in the night, and tremors after taking a pill. This has pretty much stopped since I started taking the beta blocker propranolol, unless I vary my diet.

For now I only eat chicken steaks on a roll and some chocolates. I can't take any food that's high in salts, potassium/sodium etc. Including potatoes, bananas, gravies, smoked meat, cheeses, MSG, caffeine etc.

I have to take the lamotrigine frequently, dosed with the smallest 25mg tablets, as even a small increase of its levels in my blood will make me feel high/accelerated. My dose over the past year has been 162.5mg per day, effectively one pill every 3 hours 42 minutes. If I increase the dose to 175mg per day I start to become obsessed with porn. At 200 mg I sit at my computer all day long masturbating.

My biggest problem on the lower dose has been anxiety, triggered by food intake. On only consuming the blandest foods this was almost manageable... Having recently been introduced to propranolol this anxiety has significantly reduced, and I found myself able to reduce the lamotrigine dose to 150mg per day. The anxiety fell significantly, my face stopped stinging, which it would after almost every meal on the higher dose, and I felt relaxed. On the negative side, on the lower dose, I feel nauseous most of the day, and particularly after taking a pill.

Although things are much better now than they were pre-propranolol, I'm very concerned that these side effects are worsening with time. For now I have to rise four times each night to take pills, I'd give anything to not be forced into such regimented pill taking. It seems my life revolves around taking drugs. I want some freedom.

I was previously very concerned about coming off lamotrigine as I started taking the drug in an attempt to manage the severe anxiety brought on by Keppra. However having come off Keppra and introduced propranolol I'm confident anxiety is no longer a major issue. In effect I could continue for now with the lamotrigine together with propranolol with fairly limited side effects, other than the nausea, but my diet would be limited to chicken steaks, and cups of tea.

I'm hoping you can find a drug for me that will control my epilepsy and significantly reduce these side effects, allowing me to eat a healthy diet and take the drug less often so I get a full night's sleep.

As you can see the writing is muddled, my understanding of the foods I could eat is confused, there's no reference to panic attacks when driving for fear of losing my licence, and I barely mention porn, having become afraid there was something wrong with me and it was nothing to do with the drugs. But luckily, I said enough, and he offered to put me on a relatively new drug called Fycompa, asking to keep the letter I'd written to justify this change.

On making the switch from lamotrigine to Fycompa, in less than a month, the perversion stopped completely.

In my defence, I would submit that if someone whose drink is spiked with a date-rape drug is not responsible for "letting themselves be raped", then I was not responsible for what happened here. My point being: doctors are not deemed to be responsible because there is no malicious intent, they are simply trying to help. But that's just not good enough. Doctors should not be allowed to prescribe such potent, and it would seem barely understood, drugs, without adequate protocol in place to ensure there is no harm done. To complete the metaphor: given the choice of being date-raped by a male, or spending another four years on lamotrigine, I would choose rape.

FYCOMPA

On the initial 4mg dose of Fycompa, I didn't really like anyone, even my own family. Instead, I spent all my time with McGee, sticking exactly to the recommended (months old) x 5 mins of walking, twice a day, for her first year. Though this seemed very little, vets say it's important for Labs (a breed prone to arthritis in old age), protecting their joints as they grow. As it turned out, this slow progression suited me well, for I was weak and unfit because of the beta blockers. We walked from the car park halfway up the East Lomond hill – a little further each day – and after six backbreaking months, we'd conquered the beast (three-quarters of a mile at most).

When returning from the Dick Vet Small Animal Hospital, we decided to put Bobby on steroids for six weeks in the hope that might cure the condition; at the same time, letting me test her on various foods to establish what she could and could not eat. I found that, even on steroids, she was allergic to beef, lamb, eggs, chicken, poultry, pork, basa fish, tuna, cabbage and rice, meaning she could only take one of the diets offered by the Tails online dog food company, that being a salmon kibble. Much as Bobby loved this, we kept finding other biscuits in the mix which gave her a bad reaction each time.

Deciding to create my own diet for Bobby, I took a trip to Downfield deer farm near Cupar, where Bob had just built a slaughterhouse and butchery. When telling him about Bobby's condition, he was fantastic, giving me off-cut venison meat very cheap and, more importantly – washing stomachs for me to grind myself, for I couldn't find fresh venison tripe anywhere else in the UK. Grinding deer stomachs was more difficult than you might think. I had to get heavy-duty scissors from Italy as it was too difficult cutting the stomachs with a knife one-handed. The smell was bloody awful at first, but I did get used to it. I burned out a couple of cheap mincers and two second-hand Kenwood chefs, with a mincer attachment, before giving up and buying a Buffalo heavy-duty meat grinder from the States, which even survived a piece of bullet getting caught in the cutting blade.

I was surprised at managing the butchering so easily as I could not kill a deer, but it seems, once dead, the deer is no more, and I'm fine with that. The diet started as venison, venison tripe, peas, carrots and tatties, for one stew, and salmon, peas, carrots and tatties for the other. In the early days, there was many a batch wasted due to errors. My first really stupid mistake was using garlic as a preservative – not long after making a month's batch, McGee became very edgy and restless. I checked online and found that vets say you should not feed a dog garlic as it damages their red blood cells, so what was left was consigned to the bin. On another occasion, I screwed up the agar-agar mix, the stew somehow expanded in the pots as it cooled overnight, and there was dog food all over the kitchen the next morning. There were a few other such mishaps, but eventually, it came right. I calculated the vitamin and mineral requirements for a dog Bobby's size, so as to make my own supplement that would exactly complement her diet. And on serving, the stews were mixed with porridge and beet-pulp to aid digestion.

After about a year, I discovered that dark-fleshed fish, such as salmon, should be eaten no more than twice a week because when digested the organic arsenic it contains is converted to inorganic arsenic, which is much harder for the liver to extract from the blood. Apparently, that's why cats fed on salmon all their lives will often die young of liver failure. This conversion on digestion doesn't happen with white-fleshed fish, so salmon was dropped for haddock. On top of that, she gets a minimal dose of joint supplement and probiotic to keep her in peak condition. In these early days, John was a great help with making Bobby's food, for I struggled with some of the heavy lifting, and he would come over to help whenever needed.

The first time I saw McGee angry was as a pup. We were sitting at Mum and Dad's, watching wolves on TV. It was almost dark outside, and I was sitting with my back to two big glass doors, facing the TV. Bobby was lying peacefully at Mum's feet when she leapt up and tore across the room, fiercely barking at the reflection of a wolf apparently running up behind me. Since that day, the only times I've seen her riled is when Tai, Dave's (the retired psychiatric nurse) lurcher, is aggressive with other males. She runs up and punches his side with her two front paws, forcing him to back off, then she makes friends with the dogs herself.

McGee has a submissive nature in that when we meet other dogs, she will usually roll over on her back and kick her legs in the air. However, though holding her on the floor with my hand on her shoulder until she stopped the manic behaviour as a pup did get her under control, at six months old I could not depend on her to come to my call or whistle. I'd tried reward incentives as was taught by a local dog training group, but she only came for the reward when she wanted that more than whatever else had caught her attention, otherwise she paid no heed. On one occasion, she raced off the East Sands at St Andrews into a car park; another time, she ran out from the back garden and was almost hit by a car; and on a third, she jumped up and knocked a small child over in the Heatherhall wood, not trying to hurt the kid, just boisterous play. Because I can't run after her and punish her immediately, so she knows what she's done wrong, I had to find a way to punish her for ignoring my commands. Though previously against electric shock collars, believing them cruel, this was my only option, so I bought one online with a range of 1,000 metres.

For six weeks, with the level of shock at maximum, because she ignored anything less, I took her to the beach each morning as this was the ideal place to train her not to bother kids. When she started running toward one, I'd whistle once, shout her name, then whistle a second time, and if she ignored the second whistle, I gave her a shock. The idea being that my whistling and shouting should be understood as a warning of something bad ahead, and if she heeded the warning and came back, she'd be fine – if she didn't, she'd get a shock. That way, there was nothing to suggest I was punishing her, and our mutual trust would remain strong – which was important as I wanted a companion, not a subordinate. This worked really well with it being used a maximum of twice a day and sometimes not at all in the first four weeks, and only once in the final two. Because she understood that I was warning, and not punishing her, our relationship was not changed, and she now returns immediately whenever I call.

I can't be sure Fycompa was the impetus for getting the shock collar but, though never using it maliciously, I was absolutely certain of my motives and convinced it was the best course. Seeing how well it worked with Bobby, I wouldn't hesitate to use one again, but I might never have tried it in the first place if it weren't for the aggression that came with Fycompa.

I have to confess to getting angry one day in the woods, when as Bobby was running around playing with the other dogs, a woman said I'd been cruel using the electric shock collar to train her – while she dragged her dog around on a lead, afraid he might run off were she to let him loose. I'm not saying restraining is cruel, but I can't imagine how anyone might argue that giving Bobby the freedom to roam and live her life to the full was an act of cruelty.

I have to mention the harbour cafe in St Andrews, for we love the place, still going there often to this day. It's an old-world wooden hut with three tables inside and a few more outside overlooking the harbour where small sailing boats are moored. Pat has run the place for as long as I've been going, and as the years pass, her grandchildren and other related youngsters take it in turn to do their stint waiting on the likes of us. More often than not, they are sitting at the corner table by a Calor Gas fire playing rummy when we arrive. This was where I took Bobby on her first outing to the beach, a place she so adores now she starts yodelling in the car four miles from St Andrews. It was here she developed the allergy to tuna, getting a plate from Pat whenever she came as a pup. She just gets a slice of bread now, not that she complains as she sits watching me with her golden eyes shining, waiting for the next morsel.

Although Bobby did not fix me, as Mum would suggest, she made a huge difference as a pillar of friendship and support while I battled to understand my drugs – where our excursions to the Scottish Highlands were perhaps most therapeutic of all.

*****

My first trip north was pre-Bobby-McGee, back in the January of my termination year at Dundee University. At that time, my body was in a constant state of shock, with adrenalin pumping through my veins all day long. The only thing that made me feel relaxed was driving fast – but I would lose my licence doing this on the main roads in the central belt, so I'd headed for the Highlands where there were no speed traps to worry about. Avoiding the A9 with its average speed cameras, instead I drove to Blairgowrie then on up through the Cairngorms to Braemar; at one point racing with a BMW Z4, getting away from him, letting him catch up and racing again.

Once past Braemar, I took a high single-track road over the hills. It was stunningly beautiful, traversing the top of a ridge of hills completely bare of life other than heather, with the odd solitary boulder lying where it had been dropped by a glacier thousands of years ago. I could see right across Scotland to the mountains on the west coast – with the sheer majesty of this scene revealing a welcome fresh perspective to my problems. I passed through Inverness and continued up over the Cromarty Bridge to Dornoch where I was lucky enough to get a room for half price in the Dornoch Castle Hotel. Feeling the heat on my face from a big log fire blazing in the centre of the lounge where I sat doing my crossword, it was a grand night – but of course, the next morning, I was back to square one after taking my first dose of tablets for the day.

Heading north, then west, over the top of Scotland, the scenery continued to entrance, not just the awe-inspiring mountains and glens, but the beautiful white, sandy beaches seeming yet to be discovered, for there wasn't a soul on them. I continued down the west coast and turned inland just after Applecross to stay at the Lochcarron Hotel for the night.

On the third and final day, I'd driven back toward Applecross, negotiating Bealach na Bà, an intensely steep, winding, single-track road that takes you right to the top of a mountain ridge where, after climbing a peak with a satellite mast on top, I could see the Inner Hebrides to the west and a panorama of mountain tops to the east – by far the most beautiful place I've ever seen, and I don't expect to see better. The following day, I headed home by way of the Nevis Ridge, a stunning drive to end an awe-inspiring journey. But sadly, it had no lasting effect on my mental health, for I continued to pump myself full of drugs day after day with no apparent alternative.

***

My second such trip was a lot more fun, in part because Bobby McGee was with me, but more so because I was off the Keppra and lamotrigine. Though still struggling with anger issues on the initial dose of Fycompa, I was considerably calmer and a much better driver for it. Once again, I drove by Braemar to Inverness, but this time headed to Garve and across the middle to Lochcarron where Bobby could sleep with me in my room at the Lochcarron Hotel. Because she was little more than a year old, the owner's male black Lab took a fancy to her, much to the disapproval of their black Lab bitch. Nevertheless, we had a fab time, again ascending Bealach na Bà, only this time taking a walk through the mountains. Not far, for I was still pretty weak, but next time we will do it justice.

Funnily enough, I had almost no memory at this time of my first trip up and so kept getting a sense of déjà vu. On driving to a very isolated spot, the road just petered out to nothing other than a stone structure containing a bright red letterbox by the side of an old stony brig; I was sure I'd seen it before, but just could not remember when. The same thing happened time and time again as we unwittingly retraced my journey of three years earlier.

My favourite place in the Highlands will remain unnamed so it is not spoilt… let's just say it's not far from Glenshee. We came across it by chance. When looking for a place for Bobby to pee, a local directed us to the walk and where to park. On leaving the car and entering through a large metal gate, we walked along an old farm track, following a right curvature up over a hill. There were sheep in the field, but Bobby was trained with sheep, so even if she did start a chase, she'd stop immediately on hearing my whistle, meaning we could continue with no need for concern.

Only once did we meet another walker. I think it was our second visit. He said there was a reasonable track across a four-mile stretch to the top of the glen, so we decided to give it a go. After about half a mile, we reached a second large metal gate, with a hill forest to our right and, on the left, a steep, ridged hill overshadowing a burn that meandered through the thick heather covering the floor of the glen. We walked past the forest and continued to follow tracks left by what I imagine was a quad bike, for this area was fenced off with high deer fencing, and there were about five deer roaming the area. The going was pretty rough, with very marshy patches and a burn crossing that would be easy for most, but a little awkward for me. All the same, I managed, though a bit wobbly on one of the stepping-stones, and we strode onward, eventually reaching the top of the very low-lying hill at the head of the glen. I stopped to take a gasp at the unexpected beauty of a spotless sandy beach at the near side of a small loch. Of course, as soon as Bobby saw it, she took off, charging down the hill and straight into the water.

There were foothills surrounding the loch, as if to hide it from unwanted attention. In the months to come, I would climb the three to the south side, the one on the right being particularly difficult, with me having to zig-zag across the face of its steep ascent. This wasn't so bad when travelling from right to left as my right arm could easily grab hold of the heather giving me a solid grip, but coming back from left to right, I would struggle to reach the heather, making balance difficult and progress very slow. Eventually, after about fifty nerve-racking minutes, we made it to the top, and Bobby could finally relax as she'd been watching over me all the way up. She went tearing across the plateau, full of fervour for what we'd find next. It was fantastic! Again, I could see as far as the west coast. It really felt like we were on top of the world as I wandered to the cairn, where I sat for a few minutes soaking up the atmosphere before heading back down. Taking a much shallower decent, down the far side of the hill, proved a lot more hazardous than expected, for the ground was very wet, making it hard to find solid footing. The only option was to do my best to keep dry, often having to meander way off course in doing so. As expected, Bobby found a waterhole to immerse herself in, coming out covered in black peat oil. Luckily, the heather had her near clean by the time we got back to the car.

That first trip to the loch had taken around six hours, given the unexpected obstacles, so the next time, I took a staff with a disc at the bottom, like a ski stick, to stop it going so deep into the marshy ground, making things a lot easier. This time, we set about the higher, but less steep, peak to the left of the loch. It looked like a mountain ridge on the south side, with a sharp, rocky cliff face, where I once saw what appeared to be two eagles fighting. Though most likely just buzzards, they were screeching in a way I would associate with eagles, from what I've seen in films. This climb was wetter for I was scrambling through the rushes where water flowed down the hill to avoid steeper, rockier climbs. At about an hour and a half up and back down, again the view was worth the effort.

On the way back, I got a great picture of four deer standing about fifty yards ahead of us on a low-lying summit. We often saw or heard them grunt as we walked through the glen; until one visit, when as we walked from the car, it quickly became clear that forestry workers had started their carnage. As we walked up the glen and past the forest, Bobby kept finding the carcasses of deer that had been shot and left to rot where they fell. I know it was the foresters because we met several English men with quad bikes on the way back – one holding a gun. Another asked if that was my car at the gate, and when I said it was, he said I shouldn't be parked there because there was a no parking sign, and they were about to fell the forest so their trucks needed access.

Back at the gate, there was an A4 sheet of paper on the fence next to the car with No Parking written in biro. We did go up once more that year, but the carcasses were still lying, and I didn't want Bobby eating the rotten meat, so we left it about eighteen months before returning to find the forest gone with the workers having left a squalor of unwanted wood at the entrance to the glen. *Much as that angers me, I will return, for it is ventures like these that keep me fit and healthy, and I love the place.*

In presenting so much detail about Bobby McGee, I'm trying to convey the considerable time and energy I put into caring for her, revealing a significant change in my personality. Before getting Bobby, I'd never committed to another being, whereas now, I am devoted to her. My rationale being that, if she has the happiest life possible because of me, my life will not have been wasted. Other than our first three months, I was taking Fycompa, and though having a fiery temperament on the 4mg dose, I was rarely angry with her. When on drugs like Keppra and clonazepam, I'd have had no interest in Bobby, being far too selfish and obsessed with my own life. I want you to see that there's a decent person emerging from under the veil of drugs.

***

I guess it's pretty clear who is top dog in our house, and this led to my first destructive act of aggression – back when Bobby was first diagnosed. We were at the woods, sitting in my car, when my brother David arrived. I told him that Bobby had an immune system disorder, caused by a parasite, and there was only one other recorded case in history – and he became angry, telling me there was nothing wrong with Bobby; it was just a simple problem that loads of dogs have. He said I should listen to him, for he'd had dogs for years and knew what he was talking about. I drove off then stopped on my way home to send him a very angry text, exclaiming that I would not be talked to like a child by him, etc., etc. We did not speak again for three years, with me refusing to attend his daughter's wedding as a consequence. All because of my inability to control my temper and let things go when on the 4mg dose of Fycompa.

A few days later, I was taking Bobby back to the car from the vets when she did a jobbie on the pavement. As I went to the car to get a jobbie bag, a Liverpudlian girl, standing outside a shop having a cigarette, started shouting at me.

"Clean it fucking up!"

"I'm getting a bag from my car," I answered, with remarkable restraint.

And she yelled, "You dirty fucking bastard, my kids play out here!"

So I put Bobby in the car, got a bag, put the jobbie in the bag, went into the shop where she'd returned to work and threw the bag at her, saying, "Go fuck yourself!"

Of course, the police arrived at my flat later that week, and although not charged, I was put on a register of people given to aggressive conduct, for three years.

A few weeks later, when lying in bed in the early morning, my neighbour, not long back from the pub, was sitting next door switching his remote from one music channel to another, as he did night after night. I banged hard on my bedroom wall, trying to get him to turn it off – to no avail. Eventually, after punching a small hole in the plaster, I got up, went to his front door and kicked it hard with my heel, smashing through the wood and destroying the bottom of the door.

"Turn the fucking music off!" I shouted. And he did.

The next morning, I drove about eight miles to the Strathmiglo lay-by and disposed of my shoes in a bin, frightened the police might be able to match them to marks left on his door. This is a prime example of Fycompa causing the initial aggression, followed by paranoia induced by propranolol's outer ring of unstable neurones. *I will explain later.*

In another instance, I had bought a pair of second-hand boots on eBay and taken them to a shoe repair shop in Perth to be resoled. The cobbler told me he could reuse the bottom part of the sole, but the middle sole would have to be replaced. The cost for the whole job would be £65 with new soles, but he could do it for £40 by reusing the current lower soles. On getting them back, within a week, the soles started to split again, so I went back to the shop and told him I needed the new soles as the old ones were already coming off. I lost the plot when he told me the price would be another £65, insisting I wasn't going to pay £105 to get a pair of second-hand boots repaired.

Turning away with boots in hand, I deliberately knocked over a shelf with polishes and other stuff for sale, as I marched out threatening to report the shop to Trading Standards. Of course, I did exactly that, and posted an awful review on Yellow Pages. I won't include it here, as though there may have been some justification in my anger, I was, I'm sure, at least partly to blame. *Earlier today, I removed the review from Yellow Pages and their five-star rating was restored.*

During these times, whenever a car pulled out dangerously in front of me, I would retaliate by overtaking and slowing right down to hold them up. On one such occasion, an irate driver followed me into a garage and came over to the car shouting and threatening to punch my face in. I told him to go for it, and he backed off, saying, "Aw no, I'm not doing it here so you can get me done for doing you on camera." At which point, I told him to fuck off. And he did.

Another time, at the same garage, a truck was parked right across the front – between the entrance and exit gates – making it impossible for those leaving the garage to see oncoming traffic and safely rejoin the road. So, I sat in front of the truck, waiting for the driver to return, and when he did, I was parked so he couldn't get out. He reversed quickly and darted out, almost taking the front wing off my car, so I followed him out, overtook and slowed to 20 mph – accelerating whenever he tried to overtake so he couldn't get past. Eventually, I drove off, happy I'd made my point, but later that day, the police arrived at my flat, saying a lorry driver had reported an incident. Though not really contesting the trucker's account, I added that he'd been blocking my exit and almost hit me on leaving the garage. Fortunately, I was not charged.

I loved climbing the East Lomond hill in the early morning. Initially, we just walked from the car park to the summit and back, but I wanted to build up my stamina, so we extended the route, going down the hill first and looping back through the car park, doubling the length of the walk. At first, the bottom half of the walk was a real challenge, particularly when coming back up, because with the slope running down to my left side, my left ankle was prone to go over on itself. But I saw this as an ideal exercise to build up strength in the ankle's tendons, and where it took over two hours to do the bottom loop first time round, I can now do it easily in forty minutes.

Anyway, one morning, Bobby and me were coming up over the hill, back toward the car park, when I saw a pickup truck with two young gamekeepers watching Bobby as we approached. When we reached the truck, one told me that my dog should be on a lead because there were nesting birds on the hill.

I got angry, exclaiming, "She doesn't need to be on a lead as the law in Scotland requires that dogs are kept under control at all times, but landowners cannot insist dogs are kept on leads."

He argued that there were signs down at the farm saying dogs should be kept on leads, and I said, "What's written on signs is not necessarily the law."

As we continued on up the hill, I imagined the gamekeeper shooting Bobby, me grabbing the gun from his hand and battering him and his friend to death with it before blowing their brains out. Whenever we climbed the hill thereafter – while I was on the 4mg dose of Fycompa – I would obsess over this delusion. A far more rational response would have been to tell them Bobby is allergic to eggs, but it would seem I was looking for a fight.

Another comparable example would be, when on 1,000mg of Keppra, in the first six months of 2011, a car swerved into my lane as I was overtaking on a narrow country road. On getting past, I stopped, got out of the car, and shouting in a fit of rage, I accused the driver of trying to barge me off the road. They were an elderly couple and seemed a bit frightened, so I went back to the car, still fuming, and carried on my way.

Aggression – the only behavioural side effect I would attribute to Fycompa – was just one of a broad spectrum of side effects experienced with Keppra, suggesting aggression is something in me that is easily triggered by drugs like these, but I'm most certainly not like this naturally.

When first changing to Fycompa, I told my parents this meant my personality would change again – I could not be sure how, but had read that the most common side effect with this drug was aggression. Recently, Mum told me that when I was on the initial 4mg dose she'd had to be very careful with what she said for fear of making me angry. It's hard to imagine the distress that must come with having a child whose personality changes with their medications, time and time again.

***

One day, when training a new part of my brain to "walk my left leg", John came along, taking video footage of me doing my best to follow mountain bike tracks in the forest, then walking the soft, dry sand at St Andrews beach to strengthen the tendons on my foot, and finally, the East Lomond hill, climbing the south-west side, a very difficult climb for me, where I had to lie on the ground and, grabbing tufts of grass, pull myself up the hill with my right arm. I was hoping to persuade those at the Royal Infirmary in Glasgow to let me help others by taking them out to do the same. Prof Hart did seem interested and gave me the contact details of their media group in London – for me to send the footage to – in the hope they would come up and help promote the project. I'm not sure if it was the futility of the idea or my lack of finesse, but they did not reply.

I also pitched the idea to another friend, now Professor Kohl, who I will call Alain, as I knew him when he supervised Charlie on his PhD back at St Andrews. Alain has seen the shifts in my attitudes and character over the past decade more than most. Occasionally commenting on my Facebook posts, more often than not to criticise what I'd written. I had contacted him some years earlier – while manic – hoping to get funding and support from Glasgow University to continue the work I'd started at Ninewells, and again now with the idea to teach others my radical outdoor physiotherapy. He was very supportive but will have realised I wasn't mentally stable enough to undertake such considerable ventures.

Thwarted again in my search for a meaningful vocation – not long after, the founder of the credit union, Bill Craik, died, and we were forced to look for a new treasurer. After a few months, we found a strong candidate (ex-RAF). He was very forthright in his approach, taking the bull by the horns and looking to completely change how the organisation was run. Though a big help in getting us a new computer network with some of the money Bill had left in his will, he eventually went too far, too fast. In transferring the bank accounts to his name and ordering bank cards also in his name, he'd stepped over a line and was subsequently forced to resign.

Eventually, I was made treasurer as Joyce, Bill's assistant for many years, insisted she didn't want the position. In the coming months, learning on the job, I prepared quarterly returns for the Bank of England with help from Joyce, Maggie and a girl called Sofia who, working for Fife Voluntary Action, was contracted by the county council to support credit unions and administer the deployment of funding to help in their development. With Joyce off to Canada for a holiday, I did an analysis of our business model and prepared a plan for a way forward, sending copies to the board members and Sofia.

Through this time, I made a number of journeys to Kirkcaldy to meet with Sophia and discuss my application for funding. Given the limited funds available and after several months of haggling with a guy called John Nugent at e-Channel Financial Systems – an internet software provider that would give our members access to their accounts online – these costs were eventually reduced to £4,000 for advertising and £8,000 for the internet software including installation and maintenance over the first three years. The long-term maintenance costs would be negotiated later, once the actual benefits had been established. The key to securing this deal – with John Nugent's reluctant agreement, given it was about a third of the list price – was that I would do the maintenance on our system myself. Sofia said my business proposal was the best she'd received from credit unions applying for funding, so it was looking likely we'd get the money and secure the deal.

On the negative side, the old-school members of the board were not enthusiastic about the idea of expanding. In the same way we had turned against the previous treasurer when he tried to implement change, they were now doing the same with me. I had a good number of disagreements with Maggie and Jim – the chairman – before it eventually came to a head. They refused to pay my full travel expenses on the grounds that I'd not asked for the board's permission to make the trips to meet with Sofia. Then there was a final altercation with Joyce. She had learnt the accounting from Bill, and though he had a perfectly valid method for completing the monthly returns, one devised for a time, pre-internet, when banking transaction data was not so easily accessed. I thought it needlessly complicated, given the technology that's available now. I won't go into detail, but I decided I wasn't prepared to work any longer as a "treasurer" who had to do as ordered by an assistant treasurer. Unable to control my anger, I stood up from my computer, lifted my folders and handed them to her, saying, "I can't work with you, do it yourself."

Joyce had been with the credit union much longer than me, I think from the outset, so I informed the board – by email – that I had resigned as treasurer because I could not work with her. Though I did offer to continue working the collection point in Auchtermuchty until they'd found someone to replace me, I received no further contact other than a text from Jim saying okay, and not to worry about Auchtermuchty as he would do it for now. *Was that a sigh of relief?* When I received my partial expenses cheque, I sent a load of flyers, I'd designed and had printed in Glasgow using funds from Sofia, to the credit union's offices.

Enraged because they had not bothered to ask me to meet with the board to discuss the matter further, I changed the standing order on my £4,000 loan from £150 to £1.50 per month and contacted the Financial Conduct Authority to report what I considered to be unacceptable financial practices employed by the credit union over the years. I was being a bastard because I hadn't got my way. Sometime later, I received a message from Maggie saying my direct debit was wrong and could I please fix it. I told her my circumstances had changed so the standing order would remain as it was. I did this knowing that there was nothing they could do because I lived on benefits – *as explained earlier for the recovery of my outstanding debts.*

At this point, I started carrying a knife – *due to a delusional (paranoid) disorder caused by propranolol (I will try to explain later)* – for whenever I saw men walking alone, I was sure they were relations of Maggie's out to get me. It's important to note that though the switch to 4mg Fycompa made me less selfish and ready to care for Bobby McGee, it also strengthened the malicious and spiteful traits that first came to light with Keppra.

Some months later, I received an email, out of the blue, from Chairman Jim asking me to come and discuss my grievances at Monday's board meeting. I was at a loss until I noticed that the email was dated from three months earlier, the day after I'd resigned. Apparently, it had been stuck in the outbox on his phone since then. I decided to tell them about my email to the Financial Conduct Authority, explaining that if they sorted the issues before any potential audit, they would likely be fine. This wasn't so much a kindness as me wanting them to know what I'd done (I cannot explain my reasoning). Maggie got back to me, saying she would tell the board, and that this was nothing more than sour grapes.

I have today restarted payments as best I can afford for now and will pay off the debt in full, starting back with full payments once my car is paid for. My apologies to the people at North East Fife Credit Union. I hope all is well with them now, for they are wonderful people, devoting their time, energy and, often, money (particularly in the case of Maggie who refuses to take even travel expenses) with no other aim than to help people less fortunate than themselves.

At around the time that I was officially made treasurer of the credit union, the mobility component of my Disability Living Allowance was cut from high to low rate in the changeover to Personal Independence Payment. I was sure the reason was that I lived on the first floor – though on the council's waiting list for a ground-floor flat, this didn't change the fact that I was managing stairs. I contacted an old friend at the council, and she told me that the only way to get a council flat was to get a "notice to quit" from my landlord.

You might wonder at my admitting to this, but at that time, on returning from walking Bobby, I was barely able to shuffle from my car to the flat because of the pain in my legs, so I believed I was entitled to high-rate Mobility Allowance. Where now I am strong and pain free, and will not apply for it again.

My neighbour told me the sewage pipe on the wall above the back garden was illegal – there being considerable leakage – so I told my landlord I wanted it fixed as it was making Bobby sick. Some three weeks later with nothing yet done, I informed him that I was suspending my rent payments until the issue was resolved. He insisted the sewage wasn't coming from my flat, and I pointed out that it is the combined duty of all the landlords for the building to maintain hygiene standards in common areas such as gardens.

Some two months on, I received a lawyer's letter threatening eviction if the due rent was not paid – but a notice to quit for non-payment of rent would not suffice (it had to be because the landlord was selling the property). So, I contacted the council, and they sent out a team to investigate. The entire building was inspected, unearthing a string of violations, including a few in my flat. If the work was not completed within a month, I was to report again to the council, and they would take further action – where the landlord's letting licences could potentially be suspended.

My landlord stopped by for a chat, and we agreed that he'd give me a "notice to quit" that said he was selling the flat – and in return, I'd pay the back rent and not make a further complaint to the council. He said that, had I asked, he would have done that from the outset, and we could have avoided all this trouble. On top of that, I stopped the standing order for his last month's rent, saying he could use my deposit to cover it; meaning, he did not have the chance to deduct for damage which, to be fair, wasn't all that bad, but I wasn't going to risk leaving it up to him. There were a few other issues with things like the broken stairwell banister – where I kicked up a huge stink – *I'm going to categorise this as obsessive aggression, a compulsion to be aggressive, where I would look for things that made me angry so that I could act aggressively.* Of course, aggression just gets people's backs up, so I can't complain about the way they reacted to this behaviour. Ergo, another apology, this time to Matt.

Within a month, I was offered a council flat in Ladybank, where I live now. It seemed ideal inside – a disabled person's flat, it has a big kitchen with room for wheelchair access (not that I use a wheelchair) – but the outside was pretty rough as it's a very old building. I accepted the offer – on being told that otherwise I'd be taken off the homeless register for refusing an offer of suitable accommodation – and did my best to spruce things up. Jock, a friend of Mum and Dad's, painted the place from top to bottom, doing a very good job (I should apologise to him for my reaction to some minor issues, caused by rising and penetrating damp) – then John and his mate, Ian, came to work on the place.

Ian has ADHD, which meant I had to keep nudging him back to work as his mind would wander to tales of gold mining in Fife – but that didn't change the fact that he was very capable when in the zone. We took out a dilapidated wheelchair access ramp, realigned the paving slabs by the house to make a parking spot for my car, and made several trips to a local quarry where we loaded the car boot with heavy-duty shopping bags filled with gravel which was used to level the rest of the yard.

Ian cut out channels in the walls to hide the HDMI cables and power leads for the TVs. We had to re-lift the vinyl in the living room, a number of times, to nail the hardboard tighter to the floor as we'd fitted it upside down and it kept bulging, *my fault*. He put up various hooks, a toilet-roll holder and a towel rail. And the end result was a pretty nifty little flat. I should add that the credit union, this being before we fell out, extended my loan to cover the cost of wood-effect vinyl for the entire flat, and Maggie put me in touch with a friend who came round and fitted the lot in two evenings for very little cost.

A little more about Ian. He is an amazing guy who refuses to register with unemployment, as were he to do so, he'd be forced to look for work, and that would mean him having to put up with constant bullying as he'd continually lose track of what he should be doing. So instead, he lives between his old car, no longer viable as a mode of transport, and dossing on friend's couches. In the night, he goes around the St Andrews golf courses, searching water hazards for lost balls – later selling his spoils to the local golf shops. This may seem a hard life, but for him, it's better than the alternative. He remains unregistered in his own country because he doesn't fit with what we expect of our people.

***

There was another headbanger, a black Lab called Poppy we met at the Heatherhall wood – almost certainly a lesbian, for whenever they arrived, with us already halfway around the wood, she would take off and follow our trail until catching up, then spend the rest of the walk kissing Bobby. Poor old Steve – a history lecturer at Edinburgh University – would arrive, hot on her heels, a few minutes later. I particularly enjoyed Steve's company, for he was a good listener, and I was prone to nervous chattering when on propranolol. I told him I might try to make and sell hypoallergenic dog food, based on what I'd learnt with Bobby, and he said it sounded like a great idea.

Having made a pitch for a vacant treasurer's position at another local credit union and not even received an acknowledgment, I was sure I'd been blacklisted, so I had to prove them wrong. With no other option, I decided to start my own "business" making dog food: The McGee Recipe.

I made food for Mum's friend Betty's mongrel, Rowan; Mum's labradoodle pup, Tanzi; and for Dave's lurcher and greyhound, Tai and Maggie. The biggest problem was, they would not take the full diet. Rowan didn't like fish or porridge, so Betty just took the venison. Tanzi was the same. And although Maggie would eat anything, Tai is very picky – so much so he refuses beef burgers and holds out for rump steak, because he knows he'll get it; meaning, Dave only took the venison as well. Betty actually did a good job of giving Rowan a well-balanced diet. Mum was giving Tanzi some venison but mostly chicken she'd cooked herself, and Dave was only giving them a spoonful each before bed, among their tuna and leftovers – where earlier in the evening, both Tai and Maggie had already been fed with whatever Dave had had for his own tea, this ranging from bacon and eggs to steak. All the same, I stuck at it, with John coming over once or twice a week to help.

Concerned this wasn't working as hoped, given none of the dogs, other than Bobby, were getting a fully balanced diet, I started making biscuits – a combination of all Bobby's food mixed up and baked in the oven. These were very popular with all the dogs at the Heatherhall wood, where I'd often see one come rushing from the distance to get its share. Though it was nice to be so well appreciated by these brilliant animals, Bobby was putting on the pounds, thanks to the extra meal that came from my pocket full of biscuits each day.

Selling biscuits to Mum, Betty, Dave and a couple of the dog walkers (occasionally). I built a business plan for The McGee Recipe and took it to Business Gateway, the same lot that had helped me with my web design project in Lochgelly. They did some research, and it looked likely there might actually be a market for this stuff, particularly the biscuits – but biscuits were not the way I wanted to go. First, because I don't believe dried food is best for dogs, and second, because they are much harder to make. In the end I gave up on the idea, because the dogs wouldn't take the complete diet, and the biscuits were way too much work. I suspect that the only way I might ever make The McGee Recipe a success would be if Bobby were to live a long life, still fit and strong in her latter years; but I very much doubt that I'll try again.

I hope you're not finding this dog food stuff too boring, for it feels that way in writing. The trouble is: much of my life has been very boring, a curs-ed quest for success and respect. Here's hoping the boring bits will make the rest seem more interesting.

Sadly, while working on this project, things became strained between John and me. I was demanding too much of his time, causing agitation which snowballed to negatively impact on his everyday life and relationships. This was picked up on by his doctors, so they suggested he spend less time with me. Though still coming occasionally to clean, he stopped helping with the dog food project fairly early on.

The other ongoing problem had been with my new upstairs neighbours playing electric guitar while practising for their gigs at local pubs. Initially, I would leave the flat, drive to a nearby lay-by and do a crossword, so as to get away from the noise because it made me so angry. I did go upstairs once to ask them to turn it down, even offering the younger one my headphones, but she insisted they would not fit in her rig, then declared that she knew the rules, and as long as it was between seven and eleven and did not last longer than an hour, she could play her music as loud as she liked.

There was no let-up, so I bought a BOOM speaker, and when next they played, I turned it to full blast, left it on top of the kitchen cupboards and took Bobby for a walk. The police were called out because I'd left it on for longer than an hour. They outlined the same rules she had, and I told them if she did it again the same thing would happen. I was simply retaliating, and certainly wasn't going to be forced out of my home through intimidation by noisy neighbours. *There's gotta be some sort of irony in this.*

After enduring a session of guitar practice the afternoon before, then being woken by the sound of two women having sex in the early hours of the morning as they returned from their gig – *where a heterosexual couple might have sex for half an hour, if she's lucky, lesbians can be at it for hours, and there's two of them squawking (an abomination that earplugs cannot silence)* – I got up early, put the music on and went out with Bobby. Of course, again, they made a complaint. On returning from our walk, I found a card from the police on my car window asking me to contact them regarding an incident. I went straight to the station in Cupar, explained what had happened, and again, there was no charge. I came to hate these women with a passion – with fantasies ranging from drilling a hole in the ceiling of my bedroom, through the floor into theirs, and piping up poisonous gas, to going upstairs with a machete and cutting their heads off. But this was more than mere fantasy, for were it not illegal, I would have killed them.

That sounds very melodramatic, so I will do my best to explain. Fycompa created a burning compulsion to avenge all wrongs, as I saw it, against me. Propranolol made me delusional and sure the girls upstairs were deliberately trying to torture me. As a consequence, if it was legal to kill people – meaning I wouldn't be punished and lose Bobby – I would have bought a gun, and the next time they started with the guitar, I'd have gone upstairs and shot them both, with no remorse. I don't think I'd have broken the law, but given my driving while on Keppra, maybe it was just as well that I had Bobby McGee.

On a third occasion, someone broke into my flat and turned the speaker off. There were smudged sock footprints on the sill of the bedroom window and the blind had been damaged, but on showing this to the police, they said there was no clear evidence of entry. There were several instances thereafter when I thought someone had been in the flat – the settings on my computer seeming to have been meddled with and things like that.

I was becoming increasingly more paranoid, so much so, that I had the council change the door lock and put lockable catches on all the windows. After finding one of the windows unlocked – I still can't explain how, as all the keys were hidden away in a cupboard – my only explanation was that keys for council flat window locks must all be the same, and someone had brought a key in with them, on my forgetting to lock the door. I had all the windows sealed with little polystyrene tabs, so that if it happened again, the tabs would break, and I'd have proof a window had been opened. I also fitted a Wi-Fi security camera so that no one could enter the flat without my knowledge. There were several occasions when the camera sensor was triggered, probably by a bang or hoover upstairs, but of course, I never saw anyone in the videos.

To make things worse still, my TV was on the blink, often switching from one channel to another, and many a time, the volume would rise right up to full, causing the set to switch off, as it could not cope with the vibration. At first, I thought this was the girls upstairs, having the same remote control as mine and doing it deliberately to piss me off. Then when it happened with them not in, together with the frequent triggering of the security camera, I figured it had to be a ghost *(seriously)*. Confirmation that propranolol not only caused paranoia but also slashed my IQ.

In a desperate attempt to show that I wasn't crazy, I reported a box of my pills stolen, having put them in a lay-by waste bin myself, thinking this would convince the police that my flat was being broken into. I told them that I had to report the "theft" because I needed them to confirm the loss in order to get a fresh prescription.

I should finish up by saying the "excessive noise" from upstairs stopped after the third meeting with the police, and we've had no quarrel since. Indeed, if it weren't true that council flats like ours have no noise insulation, whatsoever, there would likely have been no quarrel in the first place.

On recounting events from when I was on high-dose Fycompa, I was expecting to experience feelings similar to those I'd had at the time, as was true when covering the Keppra years. But rather than feeling aggression, I feel cheated, knowing that with appropriate healthcare, I would not have lost my friends or had my character scarred by these obnoxious traits.

That's about it for the lunacy, thank goodness, so I will now take a layman's look at what was making me unbalanced, and explain how I eventually found my way back to normality.

STIMULANTS

I'd had chronic pain in my liver and kidneys for a few years, and had bought an ultrasound massager on eBay – to ease the pain – while living at Westfield Avenue. I gave each a twelve-minute treatment once a month, thinking the ultrasound would stimulate new cell growth. On consulting with my doctor, she'd suggested it might just be muscles, but I was sure I knew liver pain – after the fall at Heriot Watt, an ache I will never forget. She looked a bit sceptical and said the only drug that might help was ramipril. But giving it another try, on minimal dosage, induced a partial-onset seizure after one tablet, so I had to find another answer. Thinking it might be cancer and believing that ultrasound would stimulate the immune system so destroying the cancerous cells, I continued the treatment in the months to come, and it definitely eased the pain if nothing else.

For the eight years I took clonazepam, I was heavily sedated, so would look to flood my diet with stimulants. I'd drink very strong coffee, Coke, Irn Bru and Red Bull, eat spicy foods like kebabs and Madras curries, cover everything I ate with salt, and have lots of chocolate – dark for the stimulants and milk for the sugars. By following this diet, I was able to achieve a degree of lucidity, at least some of the time, but on switching to Keppra and all the anticonvulsants thereafter, this diet was completely wrong, for now my brain was invigorated rather than sedated, and the last thing needed was further stimulation.

Along with liver pain, the "insulin shock" that came with eating sweets and chocolate – which had eased on stopping Keppra – was now worse than ever. I'd eaten at least four chocolate bars and drunk six cans of Coke or equivalent every day since giving up alcohol, perhaps choosing sugar as my substitute. But now these high-sugar foods were making my heart race, the left side of my face numb and my left eye twitch. An hour after having an Aero, a Boost and a can of Coke, I would fall asleep while doing the crossword, waking in shock shortly after, having no idea where I was, with adrenaline pumping through my body and my heart racing.

Drinks were a nightmare, as everything I tried switching to was laced with stimulants – diet drinks being worst of all. It seemed that every one had an artificial sweetener of some sort, all of which had an adverse effect. Eventually, I settled for bottled sparkling water to replace sweet fizzy drinks, and I love the stuff now.

As for coffee, having previously filled a Costa latte with ten sugars, I needed an alternate sweetener. From what I'd learnt online, and having tried a number of sugar alcohols, to no avail, it seemed that the best sugar substitute *(non-stimulant)* was stevia extract – a natural spice extracted from the stevia plant that's used as a treatment for diabetes in poorer countries. Buying from You Herb It in Greece and Natural Stevia Extract from China on eBay, I've never looked back. It is five times sweeter than sugar (two spoons rather than ten) and it tastes just as good, if not better. I did spend some time last year trying to make chocolate with stevia extract, but though not bad, when better able to eat sugared chocolate again, I gave up. But I still take stevia in my morning coffee.

I did look for alternative sugar-free chocolate bars, and there was one I could eat, made with erythritol, a sugar alcohol. But though the taste was good, it caused very loose stools, for apparently this "sugar" passes very quickly, going more or less straight to the bowel undigested.

For my annual ECG, post-heart-attack, I deliberately ate food that I knew would aggravate the troubles, shortly before going to the surgery. The young nurse doing the test got quite a shock and hurried off to get my doctor. On their return, I explained I'd eaten these foods to show her what was happening, and she agreed to do the Glucose Tolerance Test she'd earlier said was no longer used as there were now more effective tests. But of course, the result was within the acceptable range.

Unconvinced, a couple of days later, I heard on Radio Scotland that there was a new treatment for diabetes. It simply involved going on a liquid-only diet for sixteen weeks so as to shed all the excess fat from your organs, particularly the liver. For the course of the diet, I took a multivitamin supplement along with my probiotic to be sure I'd remain healthy.

The multivitamin was fine as long as I wasn't eating a normal diet, but I recently tried them again and found I was becoming tired when doing my crossword after lunch, though there was no "insulin shock", and I was a bit twitchy when falling asleep at night – so I will not take multivitamins again.

I had three whey protein shakes a day, along with two chicken cuppa soups, and upped the ultrasound treatment for the period of the diet to five minutes for each of the kidneys and pancreas and ten minutes for the liver, once every week. I figured this would encourage new organ tissue growth to fill gaps left by departing fat, while also stimulating the immune system to attack any cancer. *It's hard to say whether my cancer concerns were mere paranoia or a justified attempt to diagnose the relatively severe health issues that remained unexplained.*

The diet went well, but though feeling healthy and strong, I was still thinking aggressively. I'd get angry whenever my parents said anything unsupportive and would obsess about it for days afterward, but I could see this was irrational. Though my doctor had earlier suggested that aggression might just be my natural temperament – now that I wasn't sedated on clonazepam – I was sure she was wrong, for I wasn't like this before I started taking anticonvulsants. So I decided to reduce the Fycompa dose from 4mg to 3mg by cutting a quarter off. Within a week, the angry thoughts were no more, and on completing the diet, having lost fifty-one pounds, I was feeling fantastic, especially so because the pain in my liver and kidneys was also gone, as remains true to this day.

But there were still issues with anxiety, and on returning to a normal diet, though able to eat anything at first, the "insulin shock" returned within a few days. This was a huge blow given these attacks were by far my biggest concern, so I consulted with my doctor, and he agreed we should try increasing the propranolol dose from 80mg to 160mg. Though this seemed to be helping with the anxiety, it was making me very feeble. With my blood pressure falling as low as eighty-nine over forty-two, I was often unable to open my fly buttons because my fingers were too weak, particularly when it was cold outside.

On 4mg Fycompa, the muscles in my chest would tremble, most notably first thing in the morning, as had also been true, though more emphatically so, with Keppra. This made me think I might have Parkinson's or a similar neurological condition. Though both anticonvulsants are neural stimulants – making them the more likely culprits – it seemed at least feasible that prolonged use could induce chronic brain disease. However, to my great relief, on reducing Fycompa to 3mg the tremors are far less and only apparent for a short time after taking the pill, if at all.

I think it's worth pointing out that I only ever became fully aware of the side effects from one anticonvulsant when my prescription was changed to another (and they disappeared). At the time, with so many possible causes, and on what seemed like a lifelong quest to find a suitable anticonvulsant, I had to exhaust all possibilities before giving up on a drug. Perhaps explaining the apparent hypochondria.

***

As we approached Christmas 2018, I received a letter in the post, addressed "To Anthony". Inside was a Speedo swimsuit with a cross drawn through the letter S on the logo, in black marker pen. Given all the shitty things I'd done in the past few years, there were any number of people who might have sent it, including John's girlfriend who I thought was upset with me for having taken up so much of his time. On top of that, I was worried that someone had found out about the perversions I'd had while on lamotrigine.

On taking the package to the police, they took a statement and said they'd send it off for DNA analysis. I tried to contact the officer concerned several times in the coming weeks, and he eventually returned my calls, two months later, to say they'd not been able to find a DNA match, but were I to receive any more letters of this type, I should contact him again, and they would continue their investigation. Given my concern that it might be John's girlfriend, I decided to stop having him clean for me – for their's was a turbulent relationship, and I didn't want to fan the flames. Not really an agonising decision as I don't care much for cleanliness anyway.

BALANCING MY MIND

When I explained to my doctor why I'd reduced Fycompa from 4mg to 3mg, she said there was a 2mg tablet used for weaning people onto the drug and suggested I give that a try. I also asked if there was any way we could ease the anxiety without using beta blockers, for I was getting very weak, but fortunately, as it turns out, there was nothing. After a couple of weeks on the 2mg tablet, I started having panic attacks again while driving, I went back to 3mg, and they stopped immediately. Which is when I realised that Fycompa must be stopping the anxiety, and in that moment, I came to better understand the problem.

First, the underlying anxiety can be thought of as one side of a see-saw where the other side is aggression. When on 4mg Fycompa, my aggression was too high, meaning there was no underlying anxiety, whereas on 2mg, the aggression was too low so there was high underlying anxiety. In effect, the see-saw had switched from one side to the other. However, on 3mg, there was no underlying anxiety or aggression because the see-saw was balanced.

Which sounds great, but why was there still paranoia?

Now this explanation is entirely based on my own experience and is not drawn from anything I've read so should not be taken as fact. As I see it, the beta blocker, propranolol, starves beta cells of glucose – so they are effectively switched off – and this works well at first, because the cells that were causing the anxiety are now held in stasis. But there will be a ring of cells at the edge of the treated area that are only partially starved and so become volatile as they are getting enough glucose to be active but not enough to be stable. Consequentially, when the dose is increased, the problem is resolved for a short time, but soon, the ring moves out, and a new extremity of partially fed unstable cells is created.

Whatever the truth, this was my interpretation, so I decided to come off propranolol – very slowly this time, as I'd tried before and suffered significant heart palpitations as a consequence. Back then, I'd thought it was because my heart was weak, or perhaps damaged, but I now understood this would happen with any heart, as stopping a beta blocker changes the way it beats. On counting the pellets in a capsule, I found there were 160, so 1mg each, meaning it was relatively easy, though laborious, to make up my own supply of capsules and reduce the dose by 10mg each week.

I suffered quite severe paranoia when coming off propranolol, indeed, that's when I told the police my tablets had been stolen. To make sleeping easier, I asked my doctor to prescribe some very low dose clonazepam which really helped. But he was concerned by the paranoid episodes and "insulin shocks", so he arranged for me to meet with a consultant neurologist. By the time of the appointment, I was completely off propranolol so the paranoia was gone, and I'd discontinued the clonazepam as the "insulin shocks" and heart palpitations when falling asleep had also stopped, *as it turns out down to dietary changes* – so it was agreed all was well and I should remain on the 3mg dose of Fycompa. Within a few months, my blood pressure was back to normal and my strength returned, alleviating the pains in my legs.

I should also mention memory, for the majority of the stories in this book were lost to me when I was taking propranolol, and my short-term memory was virtually non-existent, so I worked with checklists, like: keys, money, tablets, wallet, phone and pen, whenever leaving the flat. Even then there were often times I had to return to the flat, unable to remember if I'd taken my tablets, only to find that I had on checking the pill caddy. In the year since, I've only returned once, and rightly so, for I had forgotten. It's hard to explain how much more difficult everyday life is without short-term memory – as if being stuck in a time bubble around the present, uncertain of all that has happened in the recent past.

For me, the long-term use of the propranolol beta blocker – in switching off brain cells to treat anxiety – was equivalent to amputating a leg to treat gout in a toe.

I'd also tried grinding up the 3mg of Fycompa and mixing it with xanthan gum – in the hope that would produce a slow-release tablet – thinking that the paranoia might be down to Fycompa levels falling too low, which might not happen with slow release. However, with the paranoia gone after stopping propranolol, I decided to try putting three-quarters of a 4mg Fycompa tablet into a capsule, as it was much easier, and that now works just as well. I can happily say the security camera hasn't been switched on since and the knife is back in the drawer.

About a month after finishing with the beta blocker, I attended my cousin Andy's wedding reception. It was my first social event in years, and though someone did spike my sparkling water with vodka – I won't say who – I survived the night. Though a little paranoid, as the beta-neurones hadn't yet fully recovered, I was fairly comfortable.

I remember speaking to the Fletchers, the only academics I'd known as a child. John is the vet who started the first deer farm in Britain, co-founder of the Scottish Deer Centre with his wife, Nicky, an artist, jeweller and published chef. On meeting John, I found myself trying to explain the calamitous goings on of the past few years, once again with the hope that all would soon be well.

Perhaps the real reason for writing this book is I'm tired of having to explain what went wrong. That, and the hope that I'll make enough money to rent a cottage in the hills, for I hate town flats.

DREAMS

Dreams are another crucial issue with epilepsy medications. I don't recall much of my dreams before taking anticonvulsants, as best I can say, they were not troubled. When on Epilim and Phenytoin they were perhaps more negative and reserved, but I was in my teens, a time when everyone's dreams are hard to interpret because of the turbulent nature of adolescent minds.

As for Tegretol, I really can't be sure, as my memories are so vague for those years. I do remember telling Mum I'd lost the ability to see images in my dreams after the brain surgery and throughout the years on Tegretol, but can't be sure whether that was down to the drug or the surgery. I started having visual dreams again while in second year at Heriot Watt, when on gabapentin. These dreams were excessively positive; though still very nervous with my dream girls – the one place where you should be able to live out your fantasies, and I couldn't even manage that. Of course, I was also taking dihydrocodeine at that time which will almost certainly have had an effect.

Clonazepam had a weird effect on me when dreaming. I started talking about myself in the third person *(I would imagine I was someone else talking to someone else about me)*. When I was going with Agnes, I'd often dream I was her, chatting with her friends, saying, "He's just so handsome." Other than that, my dreams were pretty negative on the 1mg dose, often finding myself lost in a labyrinth of corridors, trying to find my class or searching for my room at Heriot Watt, always with the overwhelming feeling of failure. Then later, on the higher 1.5mg dose, everything changed, for now I could control my dreams, making them far more enjoyable, indeed better than being awake.

Keppra was a step back, in that the dreams were the same as those on the lower 1mg dose of clonazepam, only much more severe. I'd often find myself being chased through the corridors by dark shadows, very frightening, perhaps explaining why I slept so little on Keppra. On adding lamotrigine to the pot, the dreams became very sexual, both sadistic and masochistic. On reflection, this was most certainly the closest I came to outright madness. On switching to lamotrigine alone, there was less negativity, and my dreams were little more than a sequence of insane orgasms.

Finally, to Fycompa, perhaps most interesting of all, because this is the only medication for which I monitored the effects of what I was eating. With the higher 4mg dose, my dreams were very aggressive and violent but not frightening at all. I suspect a reflection of how a professional soldier might be naturally. We think of soldiers as incredibly brave people who overcome their fears to protect us, and that may be true for people who are forced into war by circumstance, but I think it's different for the professional as they are naturally more aggressive and don't feel fear in the way an average person does. Kamikaze pilots are the perfect example – I suspect not coincidentally – coming from Japan where Fycompa was developed.

With the lower 3mg dose, on a diet low in spices, chocolate, salt and sugars, I dreamt very little, getting a great night's sleep. However, when switching to smoked sausage, for example, I found myself dreaming more. I think something to do with the manganese that's used in the smoking process. The effects were similar with salt, chocolate, cheese and the strong spices. They were, what you might call normal dreams, but after a Chinese takeaway, I did still occasionally wake feeling haunted by the torment of failure, but nothing like it once was. *On recently switching to taking Fycompa at night rather than morning, I rarely dream, that I can recall, and these dreams are relatively humdrum.*

DIET

I won't go through the bellyful of dead ends and wrong turns taken while trying to find a diet that would not aggravate "insulin shock", as that would take far too long. Instead, I will note key discoveries and explain how I eventually pieced things together.

After three days of eating smoked haddock as part of a weight-loss diet, I began to have "insulin shocks" when falling asleep. Assuming this was caused by the spices used in smoking, I switched to unsmoked, but the problem persisted. A few days later – because of the heart palpitations when falling asleep – I'd decided to try taking a cod liver oil supplement, as the omega-3 would be good for my heart. But rather than helping, the heart palpitations got much worse and the "insulin shocks" returned. The obvious conclusion was that omega-3 must be causing all of the symptoms – because it's a neural stimulant – explaining why I could not eat fish *(it's possible that vitamin D was also a factor as I've had similar reactions when taking vitamin D3 supplements).* I'd had the same issues with chicken, and on checking found that beef has about half the omega-3 of chicken, so I switched to steak. Though fruits contain less fatty acids, they also contain citric acids, fructose and glucose, and the combined effect was much the same as with foods high in omega-3.

I painstakingly tested the spices and ruled out all but white pepper and turmeric for frequent use. With garlic and onion proving to be among the most potent "insulin shock" triggers. I could have a spicy meal occasionally – perhaps a Chinese or Indian takeaway once a month – because it took two or three consecutive meals for the trigger elements to build up in my body. But even then, I'd find myself invigorated in the hours after eating. With a Madras curry, my average driving speed rose by about 10 mph, and I became more irritated by slower drivers. Perhaps explaining why the roads are so chaotic in India. Vanilla, like the hot spices, aggravated "insulin shock" on falling asleep. Ginger made my nose bleed, likely through thinning the blood, and with cinnamon, I felt faint.

Table salt, which I loved, was switched to MSG, as it contains a third of the sodium, but even this was mixed with a double measure of potassium citrate in my sauces. The idea being to increase the blood potassium level at the same time the sodium level was raised, triggering the kidneys to remove any excess sodium from my blood.

I could not take untreated porridge in the evening. I think, down to the fatty acids and high mineral content – Weetabix was even worse. I couldn't add table salt or bicarbonate of soda as they contain too much sodium, so instead, I soaked the raw oats for a few hours, adding a quarter teaspoon of potassium citrate to neutralise the fatty acids. But even then, I could only have a very small portion.

After a lot of frustration with seemingly inexplicable issues and finding that all the medically recommended alternatives made things worse not better, I eventually concocted a fairly healthy diet, while continuing to look to add variety, all home-cooked so I knew exactly what I'd eaten when things went wrong.

I should add that these adverse reactions were less after the Fycompa dose was lowered from 4mg to 3mg.

Unable to take heart medications, I tried to achieve the same effect through exercise and diet. Bobby and me walked for three to four hours every day – I'd have a chocolate whey protein shake, sweetened with stevia extract, a crispbread, Bertolli, raspberry jam and peanut butter, for breakfast; milky coffee with stevia extract and a chunky KitKat mid-morning; half a pound of beef rump steak with chips fried in olive oil and my own hot sauce for lunch; and porridge with homemade coconut/stevia ice cream for dinner. My cholesterol level was 4.2 mmol/l, my blood pressure averaged 110/60 and my heart rate was fifty-six at rest. So if nothing else, I was definitely healthier than I'd been ten years earlier.

Though the physical symptoms persisted, for the first time in four decades, my head was evenly balanced, with no anxiety, aggression, perversion, hyperactivity or sedation – better than I ever imagined possible.

As we neared Christmas 2019, I started adding turmeric to Bobby's diet to calm her immune system as an alternative to distilled salmon oil which had been making her sickly. I spoon her meat and fish stews into two small plastic jugs, spray on 3ml of extra virgin olive oil (also good for calming the immune system) and sprinkle a pinch of turmeric powder on each, then place in the microwave for two minutes. This heats the food, which is suitably cooled on mixing with cold porridge, and blends the turmeric into the oil, ensuring it is digested rather than passing straight through. Repeated for each of Bobby's two main meals in the day, this has made a huge difference. In the year since we switched to turmeric, I haven't had to give her metacam once to treat an allergic reaction, and she's become more bold – not aggressive just more confident and less submissive.

On researching turmeric's medicinal effects, I discovered it can encourage brain-cell growth, and given my beta-neurones were switched off for so long, I decided to make it the key ingredient in my own hot sauce. I don't suppose turmeric was responsible, more likely it was just cells coming back to life after having been switched off by propranolol, but in the coming weeks, I was able to complete *The Times* cryptic crossword with far greater ease than before. As we neared the end of January, I decided to finish my current book of crosswords and look for something better to do with my time, as there seemed little value in devoting my life to nothing more than solving trivial puzzles. I bought a refurbished iPad on eBay and took another stab at telling this story.

GENERAL HEALTH

I don't suppose everyday health issues are all that relevant to the Dark Veiled Faces, but they do help complete my profile, and I could do with a laugh.

The first worth mentioning was a consequence of me starting to cook my own food in an attempt to stop the "insulin shock" in the night. When living at 57 Crossgate, after cooking a tray of chicken breasts and eating two for dinner, I woke in the night with a bad stomach. The subsequent eruption of diarrhoea was the precursor to a week of trailing between bed and toilet, desperately trying to keep myself hydrated. Dad came over with some more toilet paper and cans of soup about halfway through, but nothing stayed down. Even a quarter cup of water was out the back door within minutes.

Eventually, a sample I'd left at the door for Dad to take to the doctor confirmed it was a bacteria like salmonella (I can't recall the name), but I'd already recovered by then and was, after seven days in hell, a stone and a half lighter and completely knackered. The sleep I got that night was my best ever.

The next was a hernia. When I was living at Westfield Avenue, a small lump of bowel started popping out just above the pelvic bone. If I pushed it back in, it felt fine, but it soon popped out again. Having seen Joey with a similar problem on *Friends*, I was off to the doctor, and later to the Victoria Hospital in Kirkcaldy to have the peritoneum repaired. Though tender for about a year afterward, it eventually healed completely.

And then, piles. After my doctor took a wee peek, I was off to Ninewells for a colonoscopy, which was bloody sore by the way – not the tube up the anal orifice, but the air they kept pumping in to open up the bowel so they could see what they were doing. They discovered and put elastic bands on three polyps. Enough humiliation to ensure that I now go to the toilet when the need arises, rather than waiting in the car on the side of a hill until the crossword is done.

Each of these were pretty extreme and debilitating for short periods, but my final problem began more than ten years ago. This being the "insulin shock" mentioned earlier. *Given that I had described the symptoms to my doctors, and they'd offered no suggestion that it might be down to the epilepsy medications, I figured it had to be an unrelated, everyday health issue.* This might happen twice in the day. First, after having my elevenses, mocha with ten sugars and two or three bars of chocolate; I'd be sitting doing the crossword, maybe an hour later, and drift off to sleep then wake in shock, staring forward, having no idea where I was, with my heart really pounding and adrenaline racing through my body. And second, when on Keppra and lamotrigine, the same thing would happen occasionally in the middle of the night. Whereas, with Fycompa, it happened just after falling asleep, almost every night.

I considered all sorts – from a tumour in the adrenal glands, to Coeliac disease, as white bread was among the most potent triggers (I now understand that, as well as high gluten content, white bread has a glycemic index of 75, where sucrose (table sugar) is only 65). *Although the primary triggers for "insulin shock" turned out to be stimulants, sugar supplied the energy that fuelled the attacks (the more sugar available the more severe the attack).*

Five years ago, I thought I'd found the answer but was too paranoid because of the propranolol to suggest it to my doctors. Now sure they thought me a hypochondriac, I simply explained the symptoms in the hope they would diagnose insulinoma. But of course no such diagnosis was forthcoming, so I decided to do my best to manage the symptoms with a controlled diet.

Maybe my liver had been better at restoring the blood-sugar balance when I was young, only occasionally failing to prevent the supposed insulin shock from triggering a grand-mal seizure. And though no longer inducing a seizure, that being prevented by Fycompa, I did still wake with my mind in a frenzied state of chaos, analogous to that of severe insulin shock.

The attacks would be considerably more frequent now, at least twice every day, were I not strictly managing my diet. So the options were: my pancreas was producing more insulin now than it once had been, the production of glucagon had become further depleted, or perhaps, it was just that my liver was no longer able to quickly restore the blood-sugar level when it fell too low.

Whatever the reason, there was "insulin shock" where it felt like my kidneys were sending out a blast of adrenaline to wake me up *(as they would when in insulin shock – to stop the body dying)*. The only time that my mind has been fully engaged at the outset of a seizure was before crashing the second BMW, so that is the only one I remember. My cheek and lip had felt numb a few minutes before it happened, and I suddenly felt very tired just before going into grand-mal seizure. Though increasing the dose of Keppra, and subsequent anticonvulsants – from the half dose I had been taking – prevents seizures now; I have since felt that same lip numbing before falling asleep, only to wake shortly after in "insulin shock".

Hypoglycaemia can induce seizures in people who do not have epilepsy, so I thought that might explain why I'd only ever been able to tolerate three-quarters of the minimum recommended dosage with any epilepsy medication. I did measure my blood glucose about five minutes after one of the attacks in bed, and it was 3.8mmol/l, potentially low enough to have triggered a hypoglycaemic seizure. Though I had originally believed the problem was too much sugar, when learning that anxiety can also be caused by low blood sugar, I started taking a glucose tablet whenever my lip numbed – a prelude to feeling anxious – and the symptoms did seem to ease *(I think a placebo effect)*.

I'd be surprised if others with epilepsy – certainly those who've had the troubles I have – would not give their back teeth for an alternate diagnosis. Something that could be cured or treated without these mind-altering drugs.

When writing the first draft of this book, I decided to reread and edit the previous day's work between 4 a.m. and 7 a.m. and write new pages in the late morning between 8 a.m. and 12 p.m. This worked well until, after walking the forest with Bobby in the afternoon, I decided to read another chapter in bed before going to sleep. On falling asleep, I had a particularly bad "insulin shock". The most severe yet, it was like a massive electric shock through my whole upper body. I could not for the life of me figure out why, for there had been no change in my diet that day that might explain it. The following morning, I determined that the previous afternoon's reading must have invigorated the brain lesion, in the same way that certain stimulants and high glycemic-index foods did.

As a teenager, having had seizures three or four times after reading at night, I stopped reading in bed, with the reluctant reasoning that this would not matter – better to live my life to the full than waste time reading about other people's lives.

I wasn't sure, but I thought I might have had a piece of white chocolate late in the afternoon on the day of the bad "insulin shock". So, I decided to do some evening reading and writing, a few days later – without having had any sugar since morning – to see if the episode would repeat. A little nerve-racking, but it was the only way to be sure... There was no recurrence. So, given I'd had white chocolate before, in the late afternoon, and only experienced mild heart palpitations when falling asleep, it would seem likely that the combination of the two had triggered this unusually severe "insulin shock".

Insulinoma and reactive hypoglycaemia were the only answers I could conceive of that explained all the symptoms. Though insulinoma is very rare, it can be removed surgically, so with the paranoia gone, I decided to arrange for an MRI to be done privately to confirm or rule out this diagnosis.

After setting things in motion with Tayside Complete Health to have the MRI, they emailed me to say that on checking with Ninewells they'd discovered there were multiple staples and clips left in my head post-brain-surgery, which ruled out an MRI, as it would be far too dangerous. *I shouldn't go near an MRI machine, never mind in one.*

With no suitable imaging technology available to assess my pancreas, instead, they arranged a blood test, where I had to fast for four days, to identify an insulinoma. When the consultant called to give me the great news that the test was negative, I was gutted, for I would far rather have had a benign tumour in my pancreas than be lumbered with epilepsy. Which just left reactive hypoglycaemia which cannot be treated, other than with a carefully managed diet. *I figured maybe this level of reactive hypoglycaemia would go unnoticed in an average person, but the anticonvulsants, epilepsy and brain damage meant it was more serious for me.*

Last week, when writing, I was reminded there were a couple of days after the sixteen-week diet when I could eat anything, so I decided to have nothing but whey protein shakes one day and try eating normally the next, and it worked. By giving my body twenty-four hours to normalise all the triggers (brain stimulants, like: caffeine, omega-3, sodium, manganese and magnesium) those levels don't rise high enough after eating to trigger heart palpitations or "insulin shock". Which might seem to justify my initial instinct that my blood was not being filtered as effectively as it once had been.

ME TODAY

I spend my days working on the book and walking with Bobby McGee. Well, I did until August 2020 when she damaged her hip. At first, we thought she'd torn the cruciate ligament in her right knee, then after being laid up for a about a month with little sign of improvement, she was assessed by specialist vets at the East Neuk Veterinary Clinic. As it turned out, the cruciate ligament was fine, but a physical examination identified hip dysplasia, and an X-ray revealed a bone spur on the hip – the consequence of over-zealous play-fighting with Mum's pup, Tanzi. She's doing much better now that she's lost weight, but is still noticeably protecting the hip, so will most likely need a new one before long. I'm sure she would manage with it, as is, for a good many years, but I've spent most of my life crippled by disabilities, so you can be sure that I'll do all I can to save her that indignity. I've really enjoyed writing my story. Though traumatising at times, there has been huge reward in addressing the skeletons that have haunted me and tossing them out of my closet.

Having lived two-thirds of my life in chemical hell, there are no words to describe how good it feels to find myself again. It's as if I am twelve years old (before the anticonvulsants) with my brain thinking in the way it did then, the way it is meant to think. My sex drive is back to normal. I don't drive fast, as I don't feel the need. I rarely get angry, and even when I do, it's short-lived. And I can laugh again, able to recognise humour where I once just saw annoying stupidity.

Content with my life, though still a loner, I'm fairly happy with who I am. Having said that, the 3mg dose of Fycompa may be affecting me more profoundly than I realise. After discussing Covid19 with Ross, an old friend from my St Andrews days, I made it clear I felt we should let the virus take its natural course and accept there will be losses, isolate the vulnerable and treat the sick as best we can but not lockdown the rest of the country. Perhaps not surprisingly, Ross was irate in his response for he is immunocompromised and so at greater risk from the disease. But I was unmoved by his arguments, sticking to my guns with the certainty that society as a whole would be better served by carrying on as before and accepting the losses.

Perhaps the more disturbing truth is that, though I don't want him to die, I would not mourn his death. As I see it, we all live our lives, and we all die, so there's nothing to mourn in death. Though a much easier outlook on life, for there are little in the way of emotions to contend with, the lack of empathy would seem to suggest psychopathic tendencies. On the other hand, this might just be the real me, which wouldn't necessarily be all bad, given Ross did close by saying, "Glad to see you're still feisty." *In contrast, I know I will be devastated when I lose Bobby McGee, so I'm definitely a bit odd.*

Though I did tell David to "get up and get on with it" when he broke his wrist as a child, I'm not indifferent to those who are genuinely ill. I just cannot empathise with people who are afraid of becoming ill. As I see it, we should make the most of our lives, accept there will be hurdles and get on with it. I'm not saying this is the right way, but rather, it's the only way I could have cleared the hurdles I've faced. *I should add that I had the vaccine when it became available, probably because I have no more fear of vaccines than I do of Covid19, and I prefer to go with the odds.*

On hearing there is a post-surgical cavity in the right frontal and temporal lobes of my brain, after having the CT scan, I did some research and learnt that the temporal lobes deal with encoding of memory and language recognition, and that the anterior insular cortex (the activity centre of human empathy) is a portion of the cerebral cortex folded deep within the lateral sulcus (the fissure separating the frontal and temporal lobes). So, my difficulty with language and lack of empathy are most likely down to the brain lesion (where surgery, though probably saving my life, further impaired these abilities).

I had a dream in February 2021 where Dad handed me a cloth that unfolded to reveal plasticine men playing baseball. Then morphed into a cliff face embossed with letters that read, *I'm crumbling – brain reflections everywhere...* Though it didn't really make sense, there was a sickly, unsettled feeling in my stomach. I've worried about Bobby in the past, but never another person. Even when Mum had cancer (when I was at Heriot Watt), I did not worry – as best I can remember, I never even considered the possibility that she might not recover. I think I didn't worry because I could not empathise with her. Maybe this dream was a form of empathy. Anyway, baby steps, and Dad is fine.

STOP PRESS: On going over what I'd written here, I realised that the numbing of my left cheek and lips first started when on gabapentin – my first true neural stimulant – while at Heriot Watt, whereas the "insulin shock" started with Keppra – my first strong neural stimulant – and continued with lamotrigine and Fycompa. Not long after starting on Fycompa, I realised I couldn't take the drug at bedtime, as recommended, because that made the "insulin shocks" much worse when falling asleep, so I decided to take it in first thing in the morning instead. This past year, I noticed that as we moved from the winter to the summer months, when I rose at 3 a.m., the "insulin shocks" were less frequent and much less severe. At the time, I thought this might be a delayed reaction to reducing the Fycompa to 3mg and ditching propranolol, and that the "insulin shocks" were at last beginning to ease. But then as the daylight hours shortened on reaching December, now with a 5 a.m. start, they got worse again. So, where Fycompa's blood saturation level had an extra two hours to taper off, before I went to bed at night, the "insulin shock" was less of a problem.

Anticonvulsants can induce partial-onset seizures while at the same time stopping full grand-mal attacks, so I decided to try taking the Fycompa six hours after the last meal of the day (five hours after going to bed), giving my body time to digest the food and remove excess dietary stimulants from my blood – thereby preventing an attack when falling back to sleep after taking the pill. By taking Fycompa six hours earlier, in the middle of my night's sleep, the blood saturation level has time to fall below the threshold that would trigger a partial-onset seizure – if combined with high dietary stimulants – when first going to sleep the following night.

Pea once told me that all the clues in a cryptic crossword are obvious once you know the answer, and I guess that's true with everything in life, but I'm sure I'd have solved this one long ago were it not for propranolol switching my brain cells off.

CONCLUSIONS

Though my heart may have been damaged by the five years on Keppra, when it was never at rest, I will not take heart meds again – other than as a last resort – for I would rather die early of a heart attack while walking the hills than live twenty years longer stuck at home as an invalid. I'm pretty sure my distaste for heart medications is a consequence of the ill-advised and, I would say, unnecessary prescribing of these drugs post-heart-attack. Not that it matters, for I have a stubborn head – once bitten, twice shy.

Long-term prescription drug use can damage both the liver and kidneys, so it is possible there's an excess of salts and acids in my blood, but I think that's unlikely as it would seem the "insulin shock" and tachycardia are down to three factors: high/low blood sugar *(I don't know which)*, high dietary stimulants and high anticonvulsant levels. Where blood sugar and dietary stimulants are just incidental triggers activated by the anticonvulsants.

Since the blood/Fycompa level falls below the trigger threshold after about eighteen hours – by taking it five hours after going to bed, it is below this threshold when going to bed at the same time the following day (nineteen hours later), and not taking the Fycompa dose until dietary stimulants have been filtered from my blood prevents symptoms occurring when going back to sleep. Also, by taking Fycompa six hours before breakfast, the blood saturation *(early in the day)* has fallen below the level that caused lip numbing, eye twitching, anxiety and "insulin shock" when combined with dietary stimulants like caffeine and chocolates. I did keep the glucose sweets handy for a while, just in case, but they were never needed again.

In effect, I have spent more than a decade suffering partial-onset seizures and intermittent tachycardia, induced by the overdosing of anticonvulsants. As much as that irony beggars belief, the "insulin shock" problem is finally solved. I had my first cup of mocha in almost ten years a few months ago with no reaction other than that wonderful feeling that comes with great coffee. Having tested all the problem foods since, it is confirmed: I can eat normally again – and if that proves to be the only reward that comes from the year and a half I've spent writing this book, it will have been totally worth it.

Ideally there would be a 3mg Fycompa tablet, with a five-hour delayed release, and my life would be completely unaffected by epilepsy.

The drugs used in treating epilepsy and schizophrenia are very similar, indeed many are used for both conditions. Imagine a schizophrenic brain where the regions of the brain responsible for aggression are under-active. This patient would likely suffer anxiety as a consequence. Give them a drug like Fycompa, they become more aggressive, their brain becomes balanced, and the anxiety subsides. However, giving Fycompa to an epileptic like me, while not bothering to monitor their behaviour, might over-activate these regions and create a psychopath, or something of the like. I can only speculate that I was psychopathic, when on Keppra, and on the 4mg dose of Fycompa, but there can be no doubt that I suffered severe psychosis with both Keppra and lamotrigine, and that Tegretol, clonazepam and propranolol left me an imbecile.

Whenever I was switched from one anticonvulsant to another, the dominant parts of my brain changed, thereby changing my personality. But I did not see this change. I could not assess my new-self as my old-self to determine whether the changes were good or bad. I always think my current self is how I should be – we all do. That's why it's reckoned to be impossible for a person to see madness in themselves.

Since leaving school, my epilepsy medication has changed at least a dozen times, and there was not once a follow-up to ensure the new treatment wasn't having a negative effect – a task I maintain could only be done effectively by a psychiatrist. Given we are prepared to employ psychiatrists to ensure people like Jane are correctly prescribed antidepressants, I don't see how we can possibly justify denying that same level of care to patients receiving these, more dangerous, and it would seem, less well understood, anticonvulsants.

Recreational drugs are taken on a whim, each time creating a new high, but anticonvulsants are different. Basically, when taking the first of a new anticonvulsant treatment, you start on a new high and remain on that high – though slightly more elevated after taking a pill – until weaned off the drug perhaps years later. As such, when these drugs are wrongly prescribed, it is irrational to expect accountable behaviour. *Where patients themselves are expected to scrutinise, manage and learn to recognise the adverse side effects of their medications, while those same medications render them insane – the most basic principle of mental healthcare is violated...*

The nut can't see that he's cracked.

Printed in Great Britain
by Amazon

66276803R00119